HEALTH LITERACY IMPLICATIONS
FOR HEALTH CARE REFORM

WORKSHOP SUMMARY

Theresa Wizemann, *Rapporteur*

Roundtable on Health Literacy

Board on Population Health and Public Health Practice

INSTITUTE OF MEDICINE
OF THE NATIONAL ACADEMIES

THE NATIONAL ACADEMIES PRESS
Washington, D.C.
www.nap.edu

THE NATIONAL ACADEMIES PRESS   500 Fifth Street, N.W.   Washington, DC 20001

NOTICE: The project that is the subject of this report was approved by the Governing Board of the National Research Council, whose members are drawn from the councils of the National Academy of Sciences, the National Academy of Engineering, and the Institute of Medicine.

This study was supported by contracts between the National Academy of Sciences and the Agency for Healthcare Research and Quality (HHSP233200900537P), Health Resources and Services Administration (HHSH25034004T), Association of Health Insurance Plans, American College of Physicians Foundation, GlaxoSmithKline, Johnson & Johnson, Kaiser Permanente, Merck and Co., Inc., and the Missouri Foundation for Health (09-0290-HL-09). Any opinions, findings, conclusions, or recommendations expressed in this publication are those of the author(s) and do not necessarily reflect the view of the organizations or agencies that provided support for this project.

International Standard Book Number-13:   978-0-309-16416-0
International Standard Book Number-10:   0-309-16416-8

Additional copies of this report are available from the National Academies Press, 500 Fifth Street, N.W., Lockbox 285, Washington, DC 20055; (800) 624-6242 or (202) 334-3313 (in the Washington metropolitan area); Internet, http://www.nap.edu.

For more information about the Institute of Medicine, visit the IOM home page at: www.iom.edu.

The serpent has been a symbol of long life, healing, and knowledge among almost all cultures and religions since the beginning of recorded history. The serpent adopted as a logotype by the Institute of Medicine is a relief carving from ancient Greece, now held by the Staatliche Museen in Berlin.

Suggested citation: IOM (Institute of Medicine). 2011. *Health Literacy Implications for Health Care Reform: A Workshop Summary*. Washington, DC: The National Academies Press.

"Knowing is not enough; we must apply.
Willing is not enough; we must do."
—Goethe

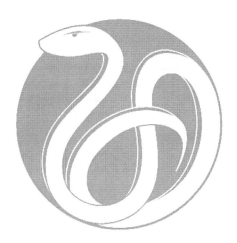

INSTITUTE OF MEDICINE
OF THE NATIONAL ACADEMIES

Advising the Nation. Improving Health.

THE NATIONAL ACADEMIES
Advisers to the Nation on Science, Engineering, and Medicine

The **National Academy of Sciences** is a private, nonprofit, self-perpetuating society of distinguished scholars engaged in scientific and engineering research, dedicated to the furtherance of science and technology and to their use for the general welfare. Upon the authority of the charter granted to it by the Congress in 1863, the Academy has a mandate that requires it to advise the federal government on scientific and technical matters. Dr. Ralph J. Cicerone is president of the National Academy of Sciences.

The **National Academy of Engineering** was established in 1964, under the charter of the National Academy of Sciences, as a parallel organization of outstanding engineers. It is autonomous in its administration and in the selection of its members, sharing with the National Academy of Sciences the responsibility for advising the federal government. The National Academy of Engineering also sponsors engineering programs aimed at meeting national needs, encourages education and research, and recognizes the superior achievements of engineers. Dr. Charles M. Vest is president of the National Academy of Engineering.

The **Institute of Medicine** was established in 1970 by the National Academy of Sciences to secure the services of eminent members of appropriate professions in the examination of policy matters pertaining to the health of the public. The Institute acts under the responsibility given to the National Academy of Sciences by its congressional charter to be an adviser to the federal government and, upon its own initiative, to identify issues of medical care, research, and education. Dr. Harvey V. Fineberg is president of the Institute of Medicine.

The **National Research Council** was organized by the National Academy of Sciences in 1916 to associate the broad community of science and technology with the Academy's purposes of furthering knowledge and advising the federal government. Functioning in accordance with general policies determined by the Academy, the Council has become the principal operating agency of both the National Academy of Sciences and the National Academy of Engineering in providing services to the government, the public, and the scientific and engineering communities. The Council is administered jointly by both Academies and the Institute of Medicine. Dr. Ralph J. Cicerone and Dr. Charles M. Vest are chair and vice chair, respectively, of the National Research Council.

www.national-academies.org

PLANNING COMMITTEE ON HEALTH CARE REFORM AND HEALTH LITERACY[1]

ARTHUR CULBERT, President and CEO, Health Literacy Missouri
GEORGE ISHAM, Medical Director and Chief Health Officer, HealthPartners
RUTH PARKER, Professor of Medicine, Emory University School of Medicine
SUSAN PISANO, Director of Communications, America's Health Insurance Plans
WINSTON WONG, Medical Director, Community Benefit, Disparities Improvement and Quality Initiatives, Kaiser Permanente

---

[1] Institute of Medicine planning committees are solely responsible for organizing the workshop, identifying topics, and choosing speakers. The responsibility for the published workshop summary rests with the workshop rapporteur and the institution.

ROUNDTABLE ON HEALTH LITERACY[1]

GEORGE ISHAM (*Chair*), Medical Director and Chief Health Officer, HealthPartners

SHARON E. BARRETT, Health Literacy Staff Consultant, Association of Clinicians for the Underserved

CINDY BRACH, Senior Health Policy Researcher, Center for Delivery, Organization, and Markets, Agency for Healthcare Research and Quality

CAROLYN COCOTAS, Senior Vice President, Quality and Corporate Compliance, F.E.G.S. Health and Human Services System

ARTHUR CULBERT, President and CEO, Health Literacy Missouri

MICHAEL L. DAVIS, Senior Vice President, Human Resources, General Mills, Inc.

BENARD P. DREYER, Professor of Pediatrics, New York University School of Medicine, and Chair, American Academy of Pediatrics Health Literacy Program Advisory Committee

LEONARD EPSTEIN, Senior Advisor, Clinical Quality and Culture, Health Resources and Services

DEBBIE FRITZ, Director, Policy and Standards, Health Management Innovations Division, GlaxoSmithKline

MARTHA GRAGG, Vice President of Program, Missouri Foundation for Health

LINDA HARRIS, Team Leader, Health Communication and eHealth Team, Office of Disease Prevention and Health Promotion, U.S. Department of Health and Human Services

BETSY L. HUMPHREYS, Deputy Director, National Library of Medicine, National Institutes of Health

JEAN KRAUSE, Executive Vice President and CEO, American College of Physicians Foundation

MARGARET LOVELAND, Global Medical Affairs, Merck & Co., Inc.

PATRICK McGARRY, Assistant Division Director, Scientific Activities Division

RUTH PARKER, Professor of Medicine, Emory University School of Medicine

YOLANDA PARTIDA, Director, National Program Office, Hablamos Juntos, University of California, San Francisco, Fresno Center for Medical Education & Research

---

[1] Institute of Medicine forums and roundtables do not issue, review, or approve individual documents. The responsibility for the published workshop summary rests with the workshop rapporteur and the institution.

vi

CLARENCE PEARSON, Consultant, Global Health Leadership and Management
SUSAN PISANO, Director of Communications, America's Health Insurance Plans
ANDREW PLEASANT, Health Literacy and Research Director, Canyon Ranch Institute
SCOTT C. RATZAN, Vice President, Global Health, Johnson & Johnson
WILL ROSS, Associate Dean for Diversity, Associate Professor of Medicine, Washington University School of Medicine
PAUL M. SCHYVE, Senior Vice President, The Joint Commission
PATRICK WAYTE, Vice President, Marketing and Health Education, American Heart Association
WINSTON F. WONG, Medical Director, Community Benefit, Disparities Improvement and Quality Initiatives, Kaiser Permanente

Study Staff

LYLA M. HERNANDEZ, Staff Director
SUZANNE LANDI, Senior Project Assistant (until November 1, 2010)
ANGELA MARTIN, Senior Project Assistant (beginning November 1, 2010)
ROSE MARIE MARTINEZ, Director, Board on Population Health and Public Health Practice

Reviewers

This report has been reviewed in draft form by individuals chosen for their diverse perspectives and technical expertise, in accordance with procedures approved by the National Research Council's Report Review Committee. The purpose of this independent review is to provide candid and critical comments that will assist the institution in making its published report as sound as possible and to ensure that the report meets institutional standards for objectivity, evidence, and responsiveness to the study charge. The review comments and draft manuscript remain confidential to protect the integrity of the process. We wish to thank the following individuals for their review of this report:

Robert Logan, National Library of Medicine
Rima Rudd, Harvard School of Public Health
Steven Rush, United Health Group Alliances
Paula Simpson, Center for Health Literacy

Although the reviewers listed above have provided many constructive comments and suggestions, they were not asked to endorse the final draft of the report before its release. The review of this report was overseen by **Hugh Tilson,** University of North Carolina School of Public Health. Appointed by the Institute of Medicine, he was responsible for making certain that an independent examination of this report was carried out in accordance with institutional procedures and that all review comments were carefully considered. Responsibility for the final content of this report rests entirely with the rapporteur and the institution.

Acknowledgments

The support of the sponsors of the Institute of Medicine Roundtable on Health Literacy made it possible to plan and conduct the workshop on the implications of health literacy for health care reform that this report summarizes. Sponsors from the Department of Health and Human Services are the Agency for Healthcare Research and Quality and the Health Resources and Services Administration. Non-federal sponsorship is provided by the Association of Health Insurance Plans, the American College of Physicians Foundation, GlaxoSmithKline, Johnson & Johnson, Kaiser Permanente, Merck and Co., Inc., and the Missouri Foundation for Health.

The roundtable thanks Stephen A. Somers and Roopa Mahadvan for preparing a commissioned paper that carefully and expertly analyzed ways in which health literacy could contribute to implementation of the provisions of the Patient Protection and Affordable Care Act. This paper provided a basis for the presentations of the other speakers. The roundtable also wishes to thank the workshop speakers whose excellent presentations generated lively discussion. These speakers were: Cheryl Bettigole, Harold Fallon, Frank Funderburk, Gerald K. McEvoy, Anand K. Parekh, Susan Pisano, Lee Sanders, and Sara Hudson Scholle.

The roundtable also wishes to thank the workshop planning committee members for their hard work in putting together a fascinating and stimulating agenda. Members of the workshop planning committee were: Arthur Culbert, George Isham, Ruth Parker, Susan Pisano, and Winston Wong.

Contents

FIGURES

BOXES

1

Introduction

On March 23, 2010, President Obama signed into law the Patient Protection and Affordable Care Act (PPACA, Public Law 111-148).[1] The PPACA was amended by the Health Care and Education Reconciliation Act of 2010 (Public Law 111-152)[2] on March 30, 2010, and the final version is referred to as the Affordable Care Act (ACA). Implementation of the Act, in concert with other major health policy initiatives of 2010, will result in significant changes to the U.S. health care system. Among its many provisions, the ACA will extend access to health care coverage to millions of Americans who have been previously uninsured. Coverage will be achieved through a variety of mechanisms including, for example, expansion of Medicaid eligibility, and the establishment of state health insurance exchanges. Many of the newly eligible individuals who should benefit most from the ACA, however, are least prepared to realize those benefits as a result of low health literacy.

Nearly 90 million adults in the United States have limited health literacy. While poor health literacy spans all demographics (sex, race, age, income, education, ability/disability, national origin/primary language, etc.), rates of low health literacy are disproportionately higher among those with lower socioeconomic status, limited education, or limited English proficiency, as well as among the elderly and individuals with mental

---

[1] Full text online at http://origin.www.gpo.gov:80/fdsys/pkg/PLAW-111publ148/pdf/PLAW-111publ148.pdf. (accessed May 1, 2011).

[2] Full text online at http://origin.www.gpo.gov:80/fdsys/pkg/PLAW-111publ152/pdf/PLAW-111publ152.pdf (accessed May 1, 2011).

or physical disabilities. Studies have shown that there is a correlation between low health literacy and poor health outcomes (Berkman et al., 2004). People with poor health literacy are more likely to make errors with their medication, less likely to complete medical treatments, more likely to be hospitalized, and have trouble navigating the health care system (IOM, 2004).

Many individuals with low health literacy will face significant challenges understanding what coverage they are eligible for under the ACA, making informed choices about the best options for themselves and their families, and completing the enrollment process. In addition to the need to attend to the health literacy of individuals, it is recognized that health literacy efforts must also address the demands and complexities of the health care systems with which patients interact. The reality is that the goals of the ACA cannot be achieved without addressing both types of health literacy issues. While the ACA contains only very limited direct mention of health literacy, there are numerous provisions where health literacy could be included in broader efforts such as expanding coverage, patient-centered care, or improving quality.

On November 10, 2010, the Institute of Medicine (IOM) Roundtable on Health Literacy convened a workshop to explore potential opportunities to advance health literacy in association with the implementation of health care reform. The Roundtable on Health Literacy focuses on building partnerships to advance the field of health literacy by translating research findings into practical strategies for implementation, and on educating the public, press, and policymakers regarding issues of health literacy. Roundtable workshops are designed to bring together leaders from the federal government, foundations, health plans, associations, and private companies to discuss challenges facing health literacy practice and research, and to identify approaches to promote health literacy in both the public and private sectors.

To facilitate discussion at this workshop, the IOM commissioned the Center for Health Care Strategies to prepare a paper reviewing the health literacy implications of the recently enacted ACA. Panelists were provided the paper in advance, and came prepared to discuss the health literacy-related opportunities and challenges that the various provisions of the new law present.

Key findings of the commissioned review, *Health Literacy Implications of the Affordable Care Act*, are presented by the authors in Chapter 2, followed by remarks from Anand Parekh, Deputy Assistant Secretary for Health, on why 2010 was a pivotal year for national action on health literacy. Chapter 3 focuses on opportunities and challenges for individuals under the ACA, and Chapter 4 explores opportunities and challenges for the organizations implementing the law. Finally, Chapter 5 presents the workshop moderator's reflections on the workshop, and a general discussion on health literacy and the implementation of the ACA. The full commissioned paper is available in the Appendix C.

Note that this workshop was organized by an independent planning committee whose role was limited to developing the meeting agenda. This summary has been prepared by a rapporteur as a factual account of the discussion that took place at the workshop. All views presented in the report are those of the individual workshop participants and should not be construed as reflecting any group consensus.

2

Health Literacy and Health Care Reform

Prior to the workshop, panelists were provided with a commissioned paper prepared by the Center for Health Care Strategies, reviewing the provisions of the ACA as they relate to health literacy.[1] To set the stage for the panel discussions the authors of the paper, *Health Literacy Implications of the Affordable Care Act*, provided a brief overview of their findings. Following this introduction, a representative of the U.S. Department of Health and Human Services (HHS) offered the Department's perspective on the commissioned paper and discussed why 2010 was a pivotal year for national action on health literacy.

HEALTH LITERACY AND THE AFFORDABLE CARE ACT

Stephen Somers, Ph.D., and Roopa Mahadevan, M.A.
Center for Health Care Strategies

The ACA is landmark legislation designed to increase access to health care coverage for millions of Americans. While it is not health literacy legislation, the goals of the ACA cannot be achieved without addressing health literacy issues. As Somers explained, the legislation offers few potent levers for health literacy; there is no forceful legislative language, no regulatory mandates, and no designated resources for action in this area. The ACA does, however, include several direct mentions of health

---

[1] The complete commissioned paper is provided in Appendix C.

literacy, and multiple indirect provisions where health literacy could be included in broader efforts such as expanding coverage, patient-centered care, or improving quality.

Direct Mentions

Title V, Subtitle A of the ACA defines health literacy for the purposes of the legislation as "the degree to which an individual has the capacity to obtain, communicate, process, and understand health information and services in order to make appropriate health decisions."[2]

In addition, four provisions in the ACA include direct mention of the term "health literacy":

- Sec. 3501: Health Care Delivery System Research; Quality Improvement Technical Assistance;
- Sec. 3506: Program to Facilitate Shared Decision-making;
- Sec. 3507: Presentation of Prescription Drug Benefit and Risk Information; and
- Sec. 5301: Training in Family Medicine, General Internal Medicine, General Pediatrics, and Physician Assistantship.

Indirect Provisions

Indirect provisions for health literacy fall into six major health and health care domains:

- **Coverage expansion:** Enrolling, reaching out to, and delivering care to health insurance coverage expansion populations in 2014 and beyond;
- **Equity:** Assuring equity in health and health care for all communities and populations;
- **Workforce:** Training providers on cultural competency and diversifying the health care provider workforce;
- **Patient information:** At appropriate reading levels in print and electronic media;
- **Public health and wellness;** and
- **Quality improvement:** Innovation to create more effective and efficient models of care, particularly for individuals with chronic illnesses requiring extensive self-management.

---

[2] *Patient Protection and Affordable Care Act*, Public Law 148, 111th Cong., 2nd sess. (March 23, 2010).

Coverage Expansion

Insurance reforms in the ACA will improve access to coverage for 32 million Americans through the individual insurance mandate, employer mandates, regional and state exchanges, and expansion of Medicaid eligibility. The legislation provides for creation of an informational consumer internet portal and funding for local outreach and enrollment assistance programs. However the ability of people to benefit from these reforms is highly dependent upon the degree to which the information is presented in ways that they can understand and use it, and there are provisions in the legislation that underscore the importance of this.

As of 2014, Medicaid will cover everyone under the age of 65 who is at or under 133 percent of the federal poverty level—potentially more than 80 million Americans, or one-quarter of the U.S. population. Again, the degree to which these eligible beneficiaries enroll is largely dependent on the degree to which they understand the opportunities that are being presented to them. Many of the characteristics often associated with poverty (e.g., limited education, mental health and substance abuse issues) suggest that health literacy is likely to be a significant issue for this population. While state Medicaid agencies have consumer assistance and readability standards, there are no state or federal entities tasked with monitoring or enforcing any readability standards across the healthcare system.

Equity

There are a variety of instances in the legislation that refer to "culturally and linguistically appropriate" communications as a means to help address racial and ethnic disparities. There are also provisions that support the needs of specific disadvantaged populations (e.g., residents of nursing facilities, and rural and tribal populations). While these provisions make no explicit link to health literacy, they provide opportunities to incorporate health literacy into implementation efforts.

Workforce

As the U.S. population grows ever more diverse, workforce development becomes increasingly more important. The ACA has provisions addressing continuing medical education support for providers to minority, rural, and/or underserved populations and areas; cultural competency and disabilities training curricula in medical and health professions schools; and diversifying the professional and paraprofessional health care workforce. "Cultural and linguistic appropriateness" is a frequent condition of eligibility for the workforce grant opportunities.

Patient Information

Health information and how that information is delivered to consumers are other areas where there are opportunities to incorporate health literacy efforts into ACA implementation. Provisions cover, for example, nutrition labeling of standard menu items at chain restaurants, improved presentation of prescription label information, medication management services in the treatment of chronic conditions, enhanced information around choice of plan eligibility and prescription drug reimbursement for Part D Medicare seniors, and the use of health information technology to disseminate information.

Public Health and Wellness

Public health is heavily reliant on the ability to get information out to the population as a whole, and for the population to understand it, Somers said. There are a number of prevention and wellness provisions throughout the ACA that offer opportunities for health literacy interventions, such as increased coverage of clinical preventive services under Medicare, Medicaid, and private health insurance; personalized wellness programs by employers and insurers; and expanded federal grants for chronic disease prevention and other public health issues.

Quality Improvement

Finally, some of the provisions that address quality, delivery systems, and cost of care provide opportunities to address health literacy (e.g., the provisions that address patient-centered care models ["medical home"] and care coordination). Also, the Center for Medicare and Medicaid Innovation will be conducting demonstration programs to research, test, and expand innovations in payment and delivery systems. There is an opportunity, Somers said, for health systems to demonstrate that interventions to address health literacy can pay off, both in higher quality care and reduced costs for the system.

In summary, Somers said that the ACA recognizes that patients need to better understand the health information they are being given in order to enroll in the available programs, stay well, and prevent and manage disease. Throughout the legislation there are opportunities for action on health literacy, including targeting interventions to those with low literacy to achieve improved health and reduced preventable hospitalizations.

2010—THE YEAR OF HEALTH LITERACY

Anand Parekh, M.D., M.P.H.
U.S. Department of Health and Human Services

Deputy Assistant Secretary for Health, Anand Parekh, began by describing four major health policy initiatives released in 2010 that he said reflect a collective recognition that improving health literacy is essential to improving health and health care: the ACA; the National Action Plan to Improve Health Literacy (HHS, 2010); the Plain Writing Act of 2010;[3,4] and the launch of Healthy People 2020 (see Box 2-1). Together, these initiatives place health literacy at the center of the national health policy conversation, Parekh said. As a result, more Americans will have meaningful access to coverage and healthcare services; use preventive and emergency and hospital services appropriately; manage their chronic conditions successfully; be more accurately diagnosed; and be healthier.

Parekh emphasized that HHS is committed to making health information accessible, understandable and actionable, and to partnering with others to realize this objective. Agencies across the department are working to implement and operationalize the elements in the ACA and the National Action Plan.

HHS ACA Activities

While low health literacy is found across all demographic groups, it disproportionately affects certain populations, including non-white racial and ethnic groups, the elderly, individuals with lower socioeconomic status and education, people with physical and mental disabilities, those with low English proficiency, and also non-native English speakers (IOM, 2004). These people are among the estimated 32 million Americans who will be newly eligible for health insurance coverage under the ACA. How we communicate with these Americans will determine whether they understand and use health care services appropriately. Passage of the ACA is just the first step toward expanded coverage, Parekh said. We now need to be accountable for clear and actionable communication with these, our most vulnerable citizens.

There are many areas where HHS can and will work toward implementing the health literacy activities mentioned in the ACA. Parekh focused his remarks on the four areas where health literacy activities are directly referenced in the ACA: quality research dissemination, shared

---

[3] A video clip from ABC News covering the passage of the Plain Writing Act of 2010 was shown to workshop participants.

[4] *Plain Writing Act of 2010*, Public Law 274, 111th Cong., 2nd sess. (October 13, 2010).

BOX 2-1
Major Health Policy Initiatives Released in 2010

The Affordable Care Act (ACA)
- Signed into law in March 2010
- Health literacy provisions are on the critical path to achieving the goals of the ACA; health care cannot be reformed in any meaningful way without health literate patients

The National Action Plan to Improve Health Literacy
- Launched by HHS Secretary Sebelius in May 2010
- Includes seven key goals to improve health literacy in the United States
Most relevant to the roundtable discussions:

   o Developing and disseminating health and safety information that is accurate, accessible, and actionable (Goal 1)
   o Promoting changes in the health care delivery system that improve health information, communication, informed decision making, and access to health services (Goal 2)

The Plain Writing Act of 2010
- Signed by President Obama, October 2010
- To improve the effectiveness and accountability of federal agencies to the public by promoting clear government communication that the public can understand and use
- Essentially a mandate for the federal government to implement important components of Goal 1 of the National Action Plan (above)
- Requires each Agency to:

   o Use plain writing in every covered document of the Agency that the Agency issues or substantially revises;
   o Designate one or more senior officials to oversee the implementation of the Act;
   o Train employees in plain writing; and
   o Establish a process for overseeing the ongoing compliance of these requirements

Healthy People 2020[a]
- Launch planned for December 2010
- Health literacy improvement will be measured in terms of how many health care providers make their instructions to patients easy to understand (through, for example, communication skills, shared decision making, personalized health information resources, easy-to-use websites)
- Healthy People 2020 objectives lend public health policy support to the ACA, the National Action Plan, and the Plain Writing Act of 2010

---

[a] Healthy People 2020 was launched in December 2010.

decision-making, medication labeling, and workforce development. These are areas where HHS agencies have already laid important groundwork in health literacy improvement, he said.

Quality Research Dissemination

Section 3501 of the ACA requires that research of the Agency for Healthcare Research and Quality (AHRQ) Center for Quality Improvement and Patient Safety be "made available to the public through multiple media and appropriate formats to reflect the varying needs of health care providers and consumers and diverse levels of health literacy."[5]

AHRQ is already translating systems research findings for consumers and providers in multiple formats, from podcasts and social media to interactive tools online, and developing easy-to-use guides on comparative effectiveness findings.

Shared Decision-Making

Section 3506 of the ACA requires HHS to "facilitate collaborative processes between patients, caregivers, authorized representatives, and clinicians that enables decision-making, provides information about tradeoffs among treatment options, and facilitates the incorporation of patient preferences and values into the medical plan." The ACA further authorizes a "program to update patient decision aids to assist health care providers and patients. Decision aids must reflect diverse levels of health literacy."[6]

AHRQ and the HHS Office of Disease Prevention and Health Promotion have collaborated to develop personalized decision support for clinical preventive services. The decision aid, *MyHealthFinder*[7] (healthfinder.gov), was designed using health literacy principles after conducting research with over 700 users, many of whom struggle with health information.

At *MyHealthFinder*, a consumer enters his or her age, sex, and several other additional inputs, and receives tailored information based on his or her individual characteristics regarding which preventive services he or she needs. The Centers for Medicare and Medicaid Services (CMS) is also designing language to help consumers compare plans more easily and make more informed health plan decisions.

---

[5] *Patient Protection and Affordable Care Act*, Public Law 148, 111th Cong., 2nd sess. (March 23, 2010).

[6] Ibid.

[7] http://www.healthfinder.gov/ (accessed February 24, 2011).

Medication Labeling

Section 3507 directs the Secretary to determine, in consultation with experts in health literacy, whether standardizing prescription drug labels and print advertising would improve decision making. The U.S. Food and Drug Administration (FDA) has taken the lead in assembling a working group focused on addressing the prescription drug information provisions in the ACA and will be reporting to Congress. The AHRQ Center for Education and Research on Therapeutics is already providing easy-to-use information to consumers on the uses and risks of new drugs and drug combinations.

Workforce Development

Section 5301 of the ACA permits the Secretary to make training grants in the primary care medical specialties, with preference for applicants that "provide training in enhanced communication with patients and in cultural competence and health literacy."[8]

HHS has already developed professional training in health literacy that informs the workforce development provisions in the ACA. The Health Resources and Services Administration (HRSA), in collaboration with the HHS Office of Minority Health and others, has formed a workforce workgroup to address approximately 20 cultural and linguistic competency components of the ACA, including health literacy. AHRQ has developed a Health Literacy Universal Precautions Toolkit[9] that provides guidance on how to improve written and spoken patient communication. AHRQ also has a health literacy training program for pharmacists, and HRSA and the Centers for Disease Control and Prevention (CDC) offer professional training in health literacy. CMS is conducting research on beneficiary-provider communications designed to help promote more effective communication and health messages by providers, and the HHS Office of Disease Prevention and Health Promotion is offering a number of health literacy webinars and Twitter chat sessions for health professionals.

Additional Health Literacy Opportunities at HHS

In addition to the four areas that are directly highlighted in the ACA, additional activities and opportunities are currently under way at HHS.

---

[8] *Patient Protection and Affordable Care Act*, Public Law 148, 111th Cong., 2nd sess. (March 23, 2010).

[9] http://www.ahrq.gov/qual/literacy/ (accessed February 24, 2011).

The Office of Minority Health, for example, is preparing to launch the National Partnership for Action to End Health Disparities, and one of the overarching themes is the promotion of culturally competent interventions, including health messages that are health literacy appropriate. As another example, CMS has developed a discharge planning checklist for patients and their caregivers to use to keep track of important information when preparing to leave the hospital, such as warning signs and symptoms, follow-up appointments, and medication reconciliation. This empowers individuals to improve their personal health outcomes, and reduces preventable hospital readmissions. CMS also is developing a standardized form for collecting concerns from beneficiaries about the quality of care they received from Medicare providers. And across all HHS agencies, communication products are being test-marketed with people with limited health literacy before they are disseminated.

Priorities and Collaboration

There is a strong foundation of health literacy improvement activities and expertise at HHS, Parekh said. The ACA, the National Action Plan, the Plain Writing Act, and Healthy People 2020 all offer important guidance and tools for leveraging these existing resources at HHS. One of the most important resources is the HHS-wide interagency working group on health literacy, which includes representatives from the Office of the Director of each of the HHS agencies. This working group was the force behind the Surgeon General's workshop on health literacy, town hall meetings on health literacy across the country, and the development of the National Action Plan for Improving Health Literacy. This group is now poised to help HHS prioritize the existing health literacy activities across the agencies, and spur collaborations.

Parekh said that the Assistant Secretary for Public Health, Howard Koh, is firmly committed to ensuring that ACA health literacy activities are implemented for as many Americans as possible. Dr. Koh has asked the HHS Working Group on Health Literacy to become engaged with those in the public and private sectors involved in implementing the ACA. Like other public health issues, ensuring health literacy is a shared commitment, with the public and private sectors working together toward a common goal. The working group will also work toward making the prevention information on the website, Healthcare.gov, actionable for all Americans. As noted by Dr. Koh in his foreword to the National Action Plan, health literacy is key to the success of our national health agenda. "It is the currency for everything we do."

DISCUSSION

Universal Versus Targeted Approach

A participant raised the issue of potential tension between the more universal approach that "health literacy is the currency for everything we do," and the targeted approach discussed by Somers of identifying at-risk populations and focusing resources and interventions specifically toward them. Parekh responded that these two approaches are equally important and need to occur in parallel. Health literacy needs to be enhanced for all Americans in all demographic groups, but at the same time we must realize that intensive efforts are needed for particular communities or populations where a lack of health literacy is leading to poor health outcomes. Somers added that private entities, such as health plans in particular, are motivated by opportunities to reduce costs. Their business case for health literacy efforts will revolve around targeted intervention for those that are most likely to experience better health and reduced costs associated with their care. Regardless, health literacy is often an afterthought, retrofit into programs after they are implemented. Health literacy must be incorporated at the beginning, when developing these programs.

Making the Business Case in the Absence of Enforcement

It was noted that there are no provisions for enforcement or accountability related to health literacy in the ACA. The Plain Writing Act is also without enforcement or consequences for failing to fulfill the intent of the law. The burden is on those both in government and outside of government to continue to be strong advocates for health literacy initiatives. A participant said that the HHS Office of Minority Health is working with the individual agency offices of minority health to ensure they are focusing on health literacy.

While many strategies from the federal government do not actually have enforcement provisions, a participant pointed out that the government does have the advantage of the bully pulpit. When leaders at the federal level are engaged in an issue, it gets attention. People also believe that even though there may not currently be enforcement, there ultimately will be if they do not comply voluntarily. Somers concurred about the potential impact of the federal bully pulpit. States prefer autonomy and can be highly resistant to federal mandates, but they can be influenced by the federal agenda to take up an important issue. Still, other levers are needed, and one approach is getting the marketplace to see health literacy as something it needs to promote for its own good (i.e., making the business case for health literacy as a means to reducing costs for insurers).

Moderator George Isham asked if, leading up to the expansion of

Medicaid and the implementation of the state-based exchanges in 2014, it would be possible to find or conduct analyses that demonstrate that lower health literacy is associated with higher costs and poorer health outcomes, perhaps data by state or locality to help make the business case to organizations implementing provisions of the law. A participant opined that few good examples exist of specific, targeted health literacy interventions that have been shown to impact costs. However another participant from Missouri stated that the state did an economic analysis that is, in fact, getting the attention of state legislators in terms of the business case for health literacy. He said that it is important to drive the effort to the state level. In that regard, a participant suggested that information about the ACA needs to be tailored to be more useful for people at the state level, to facilitate the transition from legislation to regulation.

It was also noted that there are other models in the health field that could help build a business case for health literacy; for example there is both quantitative and qualitative data on cost savings and quality improvements relating to preventable emergency room visits and preventable hospital readmissions. These activities, which incorporate significant health literacy elements, are not called "health literacy," however. If one were to ask health plans if they had health literacy programs, they might say no because they call these initiatives "quality improvement." Somers said that health plans should implement the Test of Functional Health Literacy in Adults (TOFHLA) to identify subsets of their population that have low health literacy; focus interventions around readability for that population; and then demonstrate that there are differences in hospitalizations and re-hospitalizations associated with that intervention. Quality improvement is important, but there needs to be specific attention to the health literacy aspect.

A participant recommended looking to the broader field of health communications for supportive evidence. The October 9, 2010, issue of the *Lancet*, it was pointed out, has a review article that demonstrates the value of mass media campaigns for changing health behavior and supporting public health.

Education and Outreach

A participant asked whether any provision in the ACA addresses involvement of the Department of Education, state or local school boards, or health education in any other form. Mahadevan responded that nothing in the legislation addresses this explicitly, but there is a provision that provides funding for construction and development of school-based health centers. A participant drew attention to the Healthy People Curriculum Task Force that is focusing on health education from kindergarten through college.

A question was raised about HHS outreach and education relative to Section 4103 (Medicare coverage of annual wellness visits providing a personalized prevention plan) and Section 4108 (Incentives for prevention of chronic disease in Medicaid) as there appear to be opportunities for health literacy components in these provisions. Parekh responded that there are a number of provisions in the ACA that provide authorization, but not targeted appropriation, including several of the education and outreach campaigns. As such, a collection of activities across the department will need to come together to achieve these goals. A participant noted that when money is appropriated to a particular agency within HHS, the department does not have total control over how that money is spent. However, health literacy is establishing its place among the social determinants of health, and health literacy efforts should be prominent. Parekh mentioned the Prevention and Public Health Fund created by the ACA, which will award funds for wellness related issues.

One of the provisions of the ACA calls for the Department to set up a new web portal where consumers can receive accurate, accessible health information. Parekh noted that healthfinder.gov is already an excellent portal that, in light of no new funding, could be built upon with assets from across the HHS agencies.

Moderator Isham referred to the Health Care Ecology Model by Kerr White, and suggested there is an opportunity for an ecology of health information or an ecology of health decisions model, looking at where people are making decisions (e.g., in their homes, in clinical settings), moving beyond discussion of specific literacy tools and measures to how people actually use them.

A participant referred attendees to the new AHRQ web-based Electronic Preventive Services Selector that is available as an app and a widget. It was also mentioned that there have been discussions about designing a contest for the private sector to develop applications that are health literacy-friendly.

Mahadevan raised a concern that throughout the ACA there are provisions that rely almost exclusively on the Internet for dissemination of information, whether it is enrollment in Medicaid and other public programs, or the creation of web-based tools for personalized prevention planning. Eventually, the issue of computer literacy will also need to be addressed. She noted that text messaging is also being used to spread health care information down to the community level, because texting is something that many people do every day, but they may not be going to health websites every day. Social media strategies (e.g., Facebook or Twitter) can also be used to disseminate information to the target audience. A participant said that there is a movement across the government promoting broadband adoption, and also a movement to foster digital literacy, and HHS is very interested in blending digital and health literacy.

The role of libraries was also discussed; for example the National Library of Medicine has a very extensive outreach program through the 5,000 members of the National Network of Libraries in Medicine, which also includes some public libraries and community health information centers. When trying to reach an underserved population, a participant emphasized that it important to have a person reach out to those communities to find out what they want, to train people in the community, and to introduce them to the information services that are available to them.

In closing the discussion, moderator Isham said that there are many new tools and opportunities. The challenge is to match these with how people in the target populations are actually using health information resources and making health decisions.

3

Opportunities and Challenges for Individuals Under the ACA

The ACA will directly impact individuals and their interactions with the health care system in many ways. In the context of the commissioned paper (described in Chapter 2 and available in Appendix C), panelists discussed the health literacy-related challenges and opportunities facing vulnerable populations in general, and children and the elderly in particular.

VULNERABLE POPULATIONS

Cheryl Bettigole, M.D., M.P.H.
Health Center #10, Philadelphia Department of Public Health

Vulnerable populations, as defined by *Final Report of the President's Advisory Commission on Consumer Protection and Quality in the Health Care Industry* are groups of people "made vulnerable by their financial circumstances or place of residence; health, age, or functional or developmental status; or ability to communicate effectively . . . [and] personal characteristics, such as race, ethnicity and sex" (Advisory Commission on Consumer Protection and Quality in the Health Care Industry, 1998). The ACA presents both challenges and opportunities for vulnerable populations. Bettigole provided examples in each of the six health and health care domains outlined by Somers and Mahadevan.

Coverage Expansion

Bettigole gave three examples of patients from her practice, people who were eligible for insurance before the ACA was passed, but who encountered barriers as they tried to obtain that insurance: A Portuguese-speaking man applied for Medicaid after a devastating assault requiring surgery. He was given application materials in Spanish. He obtained coverage only because of the social worker who accompanied him to the office. A young mother failed to obtain coverage for her children because she could not read the Medicaid application; they went without care. An African-American woman in her 50s refused to apply for Medicaid because she was so humiliated by her treatment at the local Department of Public Welfare office. She too goes without care.

These scenarios illustrate just a few of the challenges that will need to be addressed as coverage expansion is implemented, Bettigole said. In many cases, the literacy level in materials is too high for many patients. While some states have set a literacy level of sixth grade or lower for materials, she noted that many of her patients do not read at that level, or do not read at all. There is inadequate access to translated materials and interpreters. Many patients do not have access to computers or do not have basic computer skills. The new requirements for proof of citizenship using original documents is also a barrier to enrollment for many people. Families of mixed immigration status often fear applying for Medicaid coverage. And lastly, attitudinal barriers and health literacy among front-line medical staff are also issues.

The ACA does present many opportunities to address some of these issues. For example, the literacy level of materials that are used in the exchanges can be regulated, and interpretation and translation require-ments can be integrated as these materials are created. TV and radio can be used to reach low literacy populations and those without computer access. It is also important to engage groups already in the community that are trusted by vulnerable populations, to help bridge the divide.

With regard to Medicaid coverage expansion, Bettigole said that states should be allowed to relax the requirements for documented proof of citi-zenship. This would help facilitate other application methods like Internet and phone applications. Financial incentives for increasing enrollment of vulnerable populations are also needed. There is funding for community assistance programs and ombudsman programs in the exchange funding, and the availability of this assistance needs to be advertised on TV and radio, in multiple languages, so people know where to go for help when literacy and language requirements are not met.

Equity

Bettigole described a Haitian patient in her practice who has diabetes and high blood pressure. He misses his appointments at the clinic frequently, and often runs out of his medicines for months at a time. Earlier this year, he had a stroke. Because he was uninsured, he was not referred to rehabilitation (either inpatient or outpatient). Although he now has a walker, he has fallen repeatedly and his family is struggling to care for him at home. He and his family did not have the medical knowledge to ask about rehabilitation services and how to access them. They also did not have the knowledge or negotiating skills to realize that he should not have been sent home until he had learned to walk safely with his walker. Rehabilitation after a stroke is critical for regaining function. Ultimately, the clinic advocated for him and was able to have him readmitted for inpatient, and then outpatient rehabilitation.

This case demonstrates some of the challenges of obtaining equitable care. Patients from minority groups are often not offered the same treatment options as whites. Disparities in insurance status may explain part, but not all of the disparities in care and outcomes. In many cases, patients and families may not be comfortable challenging providers, even when they disagree or do not understand. Linguistic, cultural, and health literacy barriers compound the situation.

The non-discrimination provisions in the ACA provide protections for patients excluded from public or private coverage based on personal status. Bettigole also noted that the requirements for data collection on race, ethnicity, sex, primary language, and disability status will help facilitate assessments of progress in enrolling vulnerable populations. There is also a requirement for workforce training in culturally and linguistically appropriate care.

Workforce

Workforce development presents a variety of challenges. There is new money in the ACA for expansion of community health centers, which are expected to serve the majority of new Medicaid enrollees. But recruitment and retention of staff are major ongoing challenges for community health centers. In addition, there has been little attention to training in communication with low health literate patients, and in culturally and linguistically appropriate methods. Such training is not just for doctors, nurses, nurse practitioners, and other care providers; it is also necessary for the clerks who greet the patient and everyone else who interacts with patients along the care pathway.

Bettigole said that the expansion of the National Health Service Corp will help with recruitment of a larger workforce to community health centers. There is funding for scholar programs and loan repayment, and for the first time people will be allowed to do loan repayment service part time (i.e., they can work in a community health center, and also do academic medicine or private practice at the same time). Another opportunity is that training grants in primary care will give preference to programs that provide training in communication, cultural competency, and health literacy. It would also be helpful to develop model health professions curricula that focus on patient-centered collaborative care that is culturally and linguistically appropriate and addresses health literacy issues.

Patient Information

A woman in her 50s was sent to Bettigole's clinic for the first time after being in a local hospital for 4 weeks with what she said was "a bad cold." She arrived at the clinic with a single sheet of "discharge instructions" that had only a scribbled list of medications. There was no diagnosis, and no information about her care over the month. A full review of her hospital records revealed she had been admitted for pneumonia complicated by congestive heart failure and diabetes. Her physicians in the hospital were certain they had communicated these diagnoses to the patient, as well as follow-up care instructions. But she did not have any recollection of this.

Such patient information challenges are a daily occurrence at a public clinic. The system has huge gaps that allowed this woman to fall through the cracks. Handoffs from one institution to another pose a particular problem for patients with low health literacy. Currently there are no standards for discharge procedures in place at many hospitals. For many of the patients that do receive some sort of information, the literacy level of the material is often too high for them to understand.

Accountable care organizations (ACOs) offer a significant opportunity to improve handoffs because they have financial incentives to decrease costs and improve quality. Electronic health records are an important piece of this process, but they are useful only if the system allows for sharing of the information between facilities. Financial incentives can also be used to increase the use of community health workers and liaisons who can take the time to sit with patients who are unable to understand written materials and explain what needs to be done.

Other opportunities include using standardized tools to assess a patient's health literacy; teaching simple techniques such as "teach back" to healthcare workers to improve communication; and creating a clearing house for low health literacy materials screened to a very low (e.g., second or third grade) reading level, and even pictogram materials.

Public Health and Wellness

The ACA does expand coverage for preventive services, and funds expansions of community health interventions such as tobacco cessation and obesity prevention. This needs to be communicated clearly, in culturally and linguistically appropriate media, including not just print, but TV, radio, Internet, and social media as well. It will be especially important to collect data and assess the impact of these programs on the health of vulnerable populations.

Quality Improvement

Quality is particularly an issue for low health literacy populations with chronic conditions because they are at especially high risk for poorer outcomes. The accountable care organizations provide some incentives to improve quality of care for these populations, and Medicaid managed care plans offer opportunities to pilot interventions strategies for defined populations. Overall, improving communication has the greatest potential to improve quality of care for low literacy groups.

Summary

In conclusion, Bettigole said that systems for enrollment need to include multiple options for populations with low health literacy; there is no "one size fits all" solution. Funded community assistance and ombudsman programs should include the use of trusted community brokers who can help vulnerable populations understand insurance options and serve as advocates for those experiencing problems. Data collection and oversight will be critical to ensure that vulnerable populations enroll at rates equal to those of other communities. Financial incentives may be needed to ensure compliance with recommendations for culturally and linguistically appropriate care. Accountable care organizations need to be used as tools to improve patient-centered care, and teach back, or other standardized tools, should be required prior to discharge. There is an urgent need for widespread use of standardized discharge summaries to improve the quality of handoffs between inpatient and outpatient care. Success of these measures will depend on adequate training and commitment by the entire health care team, Bettigole said.

CHILDREN[1]

Lee Sanders, M.D., M.P.H.
University of Miami Miller School of Medicine

Health literacy is strongly associated with health outcomes. Low health literacy is associated, for example, with worse general health status, increased hospitalization, depression, and worse control of chronic illness (Berkman et al., 2004). The association for children is complex as it relates to the health literacy not just of the child, but of the parents and adult caregivers.

Health patterns and behaviors that last throughout a lifetime begin to develop early on as mother and child establish their bond. The life course perspective on child health and health literacy acknowledges that there are many factors that influence a child's health outcomes, including biology, environment, and the health system, as well as the family environment that is informed by the health literacy of the parents and other adult caregivers.

In four of the six broad themes outlined by Somers and Mahadevan there are child-specific charges that can be used to foster health literacy. Based on these, Sanders[2] offered specific recommendations to help make the ACA work for children in low literacy families, developed out of his participation with workgroups of the American Academy of Pediatrics and the Academic Pediatric Association (summarized in Box 3-1).

Child Health Insurance

There are at least 9 million children in the United States who are uninsured. Of those, at least 5 million and perhaps as many as 6 million, are eligible for public services such as Medicaid or the State Children's Health Insurance Program (CHIP) (Holahan et al., 2007). It is still not fully clear why many of them are not enrolled. Children of low literacy parents are at particularly high risk for being uninsured. They are also at risk for having decreased access to care, unmet health care needs, increased and more expensive usage as a result of increased ER visits, and decreased use of other preventive services. Many parents, not just low literacy parents, cannot complete insurance forms for child health insurance. Although Children's Health Insurance Program (CHIP) forms are required to be written at the sixth grade reading level, a 2007 analysis

---

[1] This presentation is based on a more extensive discussion of the topic which is presented in a paper in Appendix D.

[2] Further information and associated references are available in Appendix C

by Sanders showed that at least half of those forms were written above the tenth grade level (Figure 3-1).

There are a number of sections of the ACA (Sections 1413, 2715, and 3306) and the CHIP Reauthorization Act (CHIPRA) of 2009 that offer financial incentives to states for "eligibility simplification efforts." Sanders recommended that efforts include enforcing grade-level standards for enrollment forms; outreach campaigns tailored to low literacy and limited English proficiency parents; bundling of eligibility assessments at the time of enrollment in other maternal and child health care programs; and eligibility assessment of all children at school entry and at school health clinics.

Quality Improvement

Up to 15 percent of all U.S. children have a chronic condition or a special health care need (e.g., asthma, obesity, diabetes); however they comprise more than 70 percent of national child health expenditures (Perrin, 2002). Children of low-literacy parents are at the greatest risk for low health care quality. The family-centered "medical home" presents an opportunity to moderate these disparities by providing coordinated, culturally effective, and comprehensive care. All of the principles of the medical home are rooted in principles of health literacy, Sanders said, making information more user-friendly and easier to understand. A recent study by Sanders suggests that family language and literacy (limited English proficiency, lower education, and lower literacy skills) are the

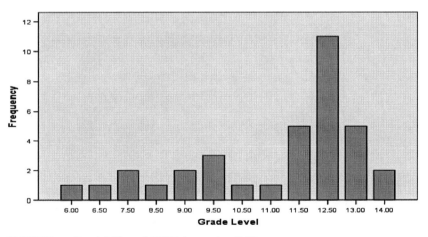

FIGURE 3-1 Readability of CHIP forms in all 50 states.
SOURCE: Sanders et al., 2007.

most modifiable social determinants of the quality of care coordination for a child.

The ACA supports quality improvement initiatives for child health, specifically: Sections 3501 and 3506 (Quality Improvement for Chronic Care), Section 4306 (Childhood Obesity Demonstration Projects), and Section 2951 (Early Childhood Home Visiting Programs).

Opportunities to improve family-centered care as outlined by Sanders include building literacy centers through the medical home; developing low literacy decision aids for children with special health care needs (including easy to use personal health records); and facilitating literacy and numeracy components of demonstration projections for preventing and managing childhood obesity (e.g., understanding food labels and portion sizes).

Child Medication Safety

There is a propensity for errors in dosing pediatric liquid medication by all parents and caregivers, but particularly among individuals with limited literacy and numeracy skills (Yin et al., 2007, 2008). Many over the counter medications do not include a dosing device, and for those that do, many have nonstandard markings on the device (Yin et al., 2010).

Section 3507 of the ACA calls for HHS to implement drug label standards, in consultation with evidence and expertise from the field of health literacy. Sanders said this provision provides the opportunity to standardize dosing instructions in both nonprescription and prescription medication, as well as to develop easy to understand dosing aids that can be used in pediatric care settings, as well as pharmacies.

The Pediatric Provider Workforce

Although the Accreditation Council for Graduate Medical Education (ACGME) competencies allude to health literacy, there are no specific requirements for it. A representative survey of all pediatricians in the United States showed that few pediatric providers use good health communication techniques, and pediatricians are asking for help in communicating across literacy barriers, not just language barriers (Turner et al., 2009). As a result, the American Academy of Pediatrics has developed an online set of training modules to teach providers about health literacy and health communication skills, including video vignettes (www.pedialink. org/cme/healthliteracy).

Sanders said that Section 5301 of the ACA can be used by HHS to make health literacy training a required component of post-graduate training, including a focus on child health and improving existing training modules.

BOX 3-1
Making the ACA Work for Children in Low-Literacy Families

To Extend Coverage to All Children:
Simplify the CHIP and Medicaid enrollment processes
- Enforce grade-level standards for paper- and web-based insurance enrollment forms
- Tailor CHIP outreach campaigns for low-literacy and limited English-proficiency parents
- Bundle eligibility assessment for all maternal and child health programs (e.g., WIC, SNAP, CHIP, Medicaid, school lunch programs)
- Assess eligibility for all maternal and child health programs at school entry and at school health clinics

To Improve the Quality of Child Health Care:
Tailor medical services for low-literacy parents of children, especially those with complex chronic illnesses
- Build health literacy through the medical home
  o Literacy-sensitive models of family-centered care, particularly for children with chronic conditions (AHRQ's Center for Quality Improvement, Section 3501; State-based Early Childhood Home Visiting Programs, Section 2951)
  o Low-literacy measures of child-health quality (Center for Medicare and Medicaid Innovation)
- Develop low-literacy decision aids for children with special needs
  o The CDC and NIH (Section 3506) should develop low-literacy decision aids for both children with special needs and their parents
  o This should include easy-to-use personal health records
- Demonstration Projects for Childhood Obesity (Section 4306)
  o Develop tools to simplify literacy- and numeracy-sensitive tasks (food labels, portion sizes)

To Improve Child Patient Safety:
Promote national standards for safe-use labeling of liquid pediatric medication
- Standardize dosing instructions on prescription and nonprescription liquid medication
- Develop easy-to-understand dosing aids for all pediatric liquid medication

To Improve the Skills of the Pediatric Workforce:
Require health literacy training
- Make health literacy training a required component of post-graduate training in child health (e.g., pediatrics, family medicine, pediatric nurse practitioners) (Section 5301)
- Improve and disseminate interactive health literacy training modules for pediatric providers

---

SOURCE: Sanders, 2010.

SENIOR CITIZENS WITH HEALTH PROBLEMS

Harold Fallon, M.D.
University of Alabama at Birmingham, School of Medicine

There are currently 40 million senior citizens in the United States and by 2020 the number is expected to reach 60 million. Fallon defined senior citizen as anyone who is on Medicare, and emphasized that there must be outreach to this sizable and growing population if we are to have a viable and healthy health care system.

Most seniors, regardless of level of education or literacy, do not understand the ACA, Fallon said. False information about what the provisions of the Act mean for seniors exacerbates fear, insecurity, and hostility, and impacts their use of the system. This is a significant and serious concern that must be addressed for all elderly, and especially those with limited health literacy.

There are generational issues to be aware of. For senior citizens, obedience to physicians' instructions is quite commonplace. Many seniors have poor science and technical knowledge, and they can be gullible, not questioning what they read in the newspaper. Privacy is very important to seniors, and their dignity often inhibits their seeking help. There is also a disinclination to entitlements. Many of today's seniors are children of the Depression, familiar with austerity and not inclined to waste money. Senior citizens also generally have an aversion to discussing disease, especially cancer, dementia, and mental illness. Poverty is an issue at any age, and compounds the many other issues seniors face.

A host of medical restrictions are more common in seniors than in younger adults, including dementias of all kinds; chronic pain, which can lead to a disinterest in life and a disinterest in seeking medical care; vision and hearing defects; and physical barriers to obtaining care.

There are the same cultural, racial, and ethnic subsets of seniors as there are for other generations. Hispanic and African American seniors have much greater difficulty entering into the healthcare system. Many of these older Americans lived through times when minorities did not have the benefits of an equal opportunity in education. Some are still not altogether adjusted to the freedoms that came during the Civil Rights era. This is something that people need to be sensitive to, Fallon noted.

What is needed, Fallon said, is a national campaign to address seniors. Every year, seniors receive a roughly 100-page document from Medicare that is an extreme challenge to navigate or understand, and Fallon suggested that many seniors simply discard it. Instead, the information needs to be brief. A succinct, one-page summary of the ACA and of Medicare is sufficient for most literate seniors, he said.

For seniors with low literacy levels, it is important to make use of all of the available community resources. The ACA affords the opportunity to expand community resources to reach senior citizens and there are a large number of senior citizen centers, retirement facilities, nursing homes, and religious facilities that provide free medical care. Many senior citizens do not use the Internet for information, and evidence suggests that television is the best vehicle for delivering health care information to seniors. Fallon recommended simple, brief, one- to two-minute TV ads.

Point of service is also an opportunity to connect with seniors. Written material alone is not sufficient, and seniors generally need more direct intervention from physicians, pharmacists, and nurses, than younger adults do. During interactions, it is important to avoid lingo and talking too fast. Politeness and respect are also at the core of successful interactions with seniors.

The electronic health record programs in the ACA also offer opportunities to improve efficiency and coordination of care, as seniors often see many different providers (e.g., dermatologist, cardiologist, internist, orthopedist).

DISCUSSION

Community Engagement

Participants discussed further the need for more community engagement. Bettigole suggested holding meetings on a local level, and potentially asking HHS to attend those meetings and coordinate stakeholders. There are multiple community groups that would like to be heard on these issues, and to be seen as partners, and the potential for funding through the outreach and assistance programs will attract organizations as well. As an example of local, community-level involvement, Sanders mentioned the Human Services Coalition in Miami, which is involved in expanding child enrollment and would be an ideal recipient agency for funds to improve outreach efforts. There is also a CHIPRA demonstration project in Florida to improve the child medical home, involving 14 primary care sites. Community programs can play a role in educating at the state level, Fallon added. There are, for example, state governors that want to do away with Medicaid and CHIP. State legislatures need to hear articulate, well-thought-out, business-like presentations on the importance of these programs for their citizens.

Enrollment

A question was asked about evidence supporting a link between the readability of forms and actual enrollment rates of children in state CHIP.

Sanders responded that there are few specific data available. The Urban Institute released a report several years back that suggested a number of reasons for the gap between the eligible and enrolled children. The readability of forms may be as much a symptom as a cause; it represents the disconnection between the overall enrollment process and the people it serves. Sanders said that there should be a state-level position that is responsible for overseeing the improvement and simplification of the enrollment process. In the CHIPRA legislation there are renewed standards that need to be enforced.

The Business Case for Health Literacy

A question was asked about what would motivate accountable care organizations to address heath literacy. Bettigole responded that a significant driver of health care costs is hospital admissions. It is in the financial interest of an ACO to keep their patients out of hospitals, and if they do need hospitalization, to see to it that they do not need to be readmitted shortly after discharge. This is a key motivator for working on health literacy, but it will take some action on the part of literacy advocates to ensure that ACOs realize this, she said.

Bettigole also pointed out that undocumented immigrants are another vulnerable population who, by and large, will remain uninsured for the foreseeable future. This fact also supports the business case for health literacy as this is a sizable population, and a hospital should have every interest in helping them avoid being admitted and readmitted due to the potential for unreimbursed costs.

Re-engineering Discharge

A participant remarked that the examples shared by Bettigole illustrate how badly hospital discharge done this country. She mentioned a study that showed that activities such as patient education and support in the hospital, scheduling follow up appointments with primary care providers before the patient leaves the hospital, and follow-up phone calls after discharge, could reduce readmissions and emergency room visits by 30 percent. The discharge process needs to be re-engineered in association with health literacy efforts. Health literacy should not be viewed as an add-on or extra expense, but a way to change how care is organized and delivered.

Sanders agreed, and noted that from the pediatric health perspective there are some good business cases from Rochester and Wisconsin that show that implementing the medical home process as part of discharge for children with special health care needs produced significant savings.

This was not exclusively related to literacy dimensions of the discharge paperwork but to the whole discharge process.

Fallon drew attention to a recent *Annals of Internal Medicine* article on hospital recidivism in the Veterans Administration health system. The study found that patients with diabetes who were discharged from the hospital and had intensive nursing follow-up, did just as well as those who were part of a "buddy group," a group of veterans who live in the same area and watch out for each other (somewhat similar to the Alcoholics Anonymous type of model). Fallon suggested that this is one low-cost way to help reduce hospital readmissions.

Roundtable Activities

A roundtable member asked Fallon for his advice on how to foster health literacy. Fallon responded that, in his opinion, what is needed is to integrate health literacy and improved communication into everything that a physician in the health care system does. The ACA, accountable care organizations, public health services, and others are all important individual pieces of the puzzle. The roundtable brings together various entities and provides the opportunity to explore ways in which integration can be achieved. Physicians need to be speaking the same language, aiming in the same direction, integrating health literacy concepts into everything they do. Sanders added that the Residency Review Committees should make literacy more prominent in graduate and continuing medical education.

4

Opportunities and Challenges for Those Implementing the ACA

In addition to the impact of the ACA on individuals discussed in Chapter 3, the new law presents a variety of challenges and opportunities for those organizations involved in implementing the different provisions of the Act. Perspectives on health literacy and the law in the context of the commissioned paper were provided by representatives of the federal government health insurer, Centers for Medicare and Medicaid Services (CMS); the private health insurance industry; a voluntary quality accreditation organization; and health system pharmacists.

CENTER FOR MEDICARE AND MEDICAID SERVICES

Frank Funderburk
Center for Medicare and Medicaid Services

There are a number of provisions of the ACA that are particularly relevant to the CMS, including:

- Supporting informed consumer decision making;
- Standardizing prescription drug information and insurance plan information;
- Improving communications with diverse, low literacy patients;
- Improving beneficiary-provider communication;
- Encouraging use of new preventive care benefits; and

- Promoting health care system innovation, which is the charge of the new Center for Medicare and Medicaid Innovation.

Funderburk's team at CMS focuses on using social marketing techniques supported by rigorous consumer testing, an approach that is applicable to both health literacy and to the ACA implementation goals.

Social Marketing

Vulnerable populations within Medicare, Medicaid, and CHIP include patients who are disabled (dual eligible) or have chronic diseases, seniors, low-income individuals and families, and people with low English proficiency. By taking a social marketing perspective in trying to reach these diverse audiences, CMS takes into account health literacy, culture, language, attitudes, perceptions, and "consumer reality," that is, consumer needs, values, beliefs, motivations, and behaviors. The goal is to identify barriers to individuals taking a more active role in their personal health care. CMS is using plain language and consumer-centered design in its products and materials, and conducting extensive testing of materials and messages. Funderburk referred participants to a recently developed and disseminated CMS toolkit for making written materials more user friendly (http://www.cms.gov/WrittenMaterialsToolkit). A campaign team then helps to develop outreach activities for both general audiences and targeted audiences. An important part of the process is evaluating the behavioral impact of the marketing campaigns, and then refining and repeating the process.

CMS is using social marketing to improve communication activities that are particularly relevant to implementation of the ACA, including communications related to discharge planning, CHIP enrollment, and understanding Medicare choices. One of the specific audiences CMS has been trying to reach is the 2-3 million people who are eligible for, but have not enrolled in, low-income subsidy. This provides them with Medicare Part D prescription drug coverage at no, or very low cost, depending on their income level. CMS has conducted extensive focus groups and individual interviews with a variety of audiences, as well as an experimental field test of direct marketing techniques, to see if the agency could achieve a measurable impact in the number of people in this target audience applying for the subsidy benefit. The data suggest that a carefully constructed CMS letter can increase the application rate for the low-income subsidy if it is written in plain language, provides very simple steps to follow, and includes the phone number of a local contact person. More labor intensive approaches, including one-on-one assistance, were not substantially more effective than the letter, and are much more expensive.

Another area of focus is the Medicare Home Health Compare website (for beneficiaries to compare Medicare-certified home health agencies). The homepage was redesigned based on the results of consumer testing and is now more interesting, understandable, and simpler to use.

Fundeburk also described a discharge planning checklist that is currently being evaluated by several quality improvement organizations. CMS has taken the specific elements of discharge planning and broken them into simple steps so patients and caregivers can read and refer to them when they are being discharged. For example, the checklist reminds them of important questions to ask, gives details about the kind of help they will be needing at home, and provides a place for notes. Preliminary tests with patients, caregivers, and practitioners indicates that this is an effective way to impart important discharge information.

As mentioned in an earlier presentation, the Medicare handbook is a very lengthy and complex document. Unfortunately, Funderburk said, most of the content is legislatively mandated, so CMS is somewhat limited in the ways in which the handbook can be changed. One way the agency is trying to improve it is by making the decision tree a little simpler. A new flow chart takes beneficiaries through a series of choices, for example: Do you want original Medicare or full Medicare Advantage Plan? If you are choosing original Medicare, do you want drug coverage? If yes, consider if you need a Medigap Plan. Testing has indicated that people are finding this flow chart to be helpful (Figure 4-1).

Next Steps

CMS is expanding into alternative communications channels and techniques, such as "edutainment," creating photo and radio novellas to engage certain populations. The agency is also looking at ways to expand communications to new audiences, working with staff and partners to help them communicate more effectively, and exploring ways to measure population health literacy. The main goal is to not leave people behind, and that means the agency needs to continue to provide materials in a written format, as well as in alternative formats.

The Center for Medicare and Medicaid Innovation, funded under the ACA, is designed to help realize the vision of an ideal health care system through high quality, reduced avoidable costs, and patient- and community-centered care. The approach looks at the health care system as a whole, with the health care consumer as an active part of the system. Health literacy will play an important role in achieving this vision. Funderburk said that the center provides a tremendous opportunity to look at how improvements in health literacy can help build an accountable health care system, and ways in which improvements in health literacy can be

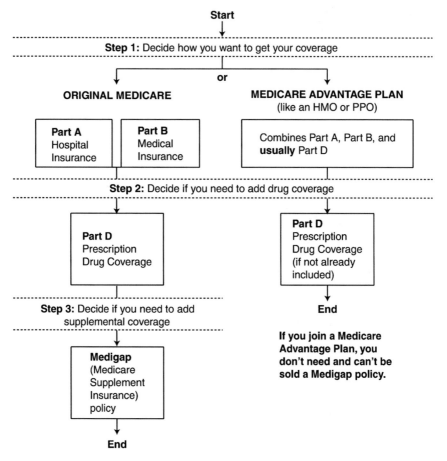

FIGURE 4-1 Flow chart simplifying Medicare choices.
SOURCE: Funderbunk, 2010.

linked to specific behaviors and patient-centered outcomes in environments like the patient-centered primary care environment. (Funderbunk noted that in testing, the term *medical home* was not well received by individuals.) Accountability for improving health literacy could also support more general health care system improvements.

In conclusion, Funderburk said that improved health literacy can help build an accountable health care system; support better consumer decision-making; help reduce avoidable costs; produce better health outcomes; and improve the quality of life of CMS beneficiary populations and the people who care for them.

INSURERS

Susan Pisano, M.A.
America's Health Insurance Plans

The ACA affects every aspect of what insurance companies do, and all of the people they serve and partner with, Pisano began. The major challenges relative to health literacy are also the major challenges relative to implementation of the ACA in general. The specific challenges relative to the health literacy-related provisions in the law are the same challenges that affect efforts to advance health literacy in general. America's Health Insurance Plans (AHIP) is a national association that represents nearly 1,300 member companies that provide health insurance coverage to more than 200 million Americans. A challenge for many of the member companies is that they are working to build and advance heath literacy programs at the same time that they are trying to implement health care reforms.

While the ACA does not specify that all patient tools, programs, and approaches should be developed using principles of clear health communication, it offers enormous potential to develop tools that are clear, easy to use, and relevant, and for the industry to learn as it goes along. For example, Section 2715 of the ACA calls for standard definitions and uniform explanation of coverage documents. Through focus groups, AHIP learned that consumers like to have a clear, easy-to-use summary, but they also want to know where they can get more detailed information. Providing that link to more information serves two purposes. One is obviously so patients can get the information they need. The other is that the availability of the information signals a level of transparency that engenders trust in the source.

One of the biggest challenges in implementing the ACA, Pisano said, is that health literacy was not a guiding principle in the drafting. What this means is that every coalition that is built and every program that is developed will require somebody to look for the opportunities and step up and take initiative. This is played out in various ways at AHIP, Pisano said. For example, AHIP incorporates health literacy into its comment letters. This may seem like a simple step, but Pisano advises her colleagues to look for every opportunity to incorporate health literacy and cultural competence into the work they are doing. AHIP is also providing tools and resources to member companies as they are developing new programs; encouraging them to take a few initial steps, bring a team together, assess their organizations, develop policies and procedures, make a plan, and train their people. AHIP worked with Emory University on the development of an assessment tool that enables health plans to evaluate if they have the infrastructure that supports good, clear communication. The tool was tested at 18 member companies, including national organizations, regional companies, and local companies (many of whom serve primarily Medicaid beneficiaries) and is now in general use. Member companies are also using different media approaches to begin to educate the populations they serve about what health care reform is, and what it means for them.

One of the challenges for AHIP is determining where to set the priorities. There are opportunities everywhere, Pisano said, such as in the direct reference to health literacy in drug labeling (Section 3507). Even though insurers are not the locus of information on prescription drugs, AHIP has an opportunity because many of its member companies use personal health records that include beneficiaries' prescription drug information.

With respect to workforce training, a number of member companies are working with their provider network, using AHIP toolkits, to encourage cross-cultural training of physicians, nurses, case managers, and health plan staff. This is an example of an area that can be built on as reform is being implemented. The primary area that member companies have been working on is how best to engage consumers and make it clear to them what their health benefits allow them to do. Companies have been developing plain language versions of benefits toolkits to support enrollment decisions, and summarizing lengthy documents in clear, one-page charts. With respect to Medicaid expansion, a number of member companies have been developing messaging and materials that incorporate an individual's cultural beliefs and attitudes about the health care system, including preferred language.

The ACA touches everything that insurers do, Pisano concluded, and these examples show just a few areas in which AHIP member companies are active. A concerted, multistakeholder coordinated strategy to infuse health literacy into the implementation of the law is necessary if we are to achieve the full benefit of health care reform.

QUALITY

Sarah Hudson Scholle, Dr.P.H.
National Committee on Quality Assurance

Health reform provides many new opportunities to focus on individuals and choice, equitable care, enrollment, delivery innovations, performance measurement, and engaging patients in shared decision making. But from the perspective of individuals with low health literacy, the ACA actually sets some relatively high expectations and new roles for consumers. It will be important to consider not just whether materials and tools are addressing health literacy needs, Scholle said, but how to get patients, families, and communities activated and engaged in this transformation.

Activated Consumers

Research has shown that activated patients are better consumers (Hibbard, 2009). The more people are participants in their own health care, the more likely they will be taking actions such as researching the qualifications of doctors, recognizing reliable health websites, using health resource books, finding comparative information about hospital quality, or comparing available health plans. These are demanding activities and low health literacy, alone or combined with difficulty understanding the language, makes it very challenging for consumers to get involved to the extent that the legislation expects or requires. People that have the lowest activation are also those with the lowest health literacy.

Scholle noted that the National Committee on Quality Assurance (NCQA) collects and reports data on quality and publishes health care report cards. Most people, however, would not know how to use them. The first step is to present information in a way that consumers can use. At the same time, it is necessary to get consumers to think that the information is, in fact, something that is useful to them. Research suggests that health literacy and activation are independent but related concepts. Scholle suggested that working on this concept of activation or engagement could help to compensate for some of the problems associated with low health literacy.

Opportunities to Engage Consumers

New delivery system approaches, such as the patient-centered medical home and accountable care organizations, have opportunities to support both literacy and patient engagement. These systems provide a locus of accountability and a place where individuals feel like they have a relationship with a trusted partner in their health care. Advances in literacy and engagement can be achieved using aspects of these systems such as health information technology, systematic approaches to care, connections to the community, and care coordination.

The NCQA has built the concept of health literacy into its patient-centered medical home program. It is expected, for example, that patients will receive information about how the practice works (e.g., how to make appointments, request medication refills). Practices should be identifying and documenting cultural and linguistic needs, and assessing family social and cultural resources and characteristics. In the process of care, tools such as medication reconciliation can be used to track patient medications. Practices should also be developing individualized self-management plans and providing clinical summaries that are meaningful to patients and their families. This also involves assessing patient readiness and connecting patients with self-management support. Practices should always be measuring and improving patient experiences. To achieve this, Scholle noted, there may be a need for new skills development for practitioners.

The Challenge of Choice

The ACA presents the Medicaid and uninsured populations with the huge responsibility of choosing a health plan. These populations in general have less experience with and knowledge of insurance. Will people know how to enroll? Will they understand what cost sharing, benefits, and networks they should select? Will they know how to choose what is best for them based on both cost and quality?

One approach to helping consumers is the concept of "choice architecture." Offer consumers an opportunity to have the exchanges picked for them. Offer high-quality, low-cost plan options and identify important plan features by person. Information could be enhanced with some sort of "seal of approval" for low-cost, high-quality plans. Quality measures should be used in setting payments.

The ACA also has requirements or expectations for new quality measures. The NCQA is very interested in patient reported measures of both their experiences of care, and their outcomes over time. The NCQA is looking at cross-cutting measures, and structural and process measures, as well as how best to collect the data, including reaching out to disadvantaged or vulnerable populations.

Research Needs

With the new Center for Medicare and Medicaid Innovation, the NCQA envisions opportunities to address issues around activating patients, providing them with simple information, and giving them the support they need to be involved in self-care decision making. The NCQA also hopes to gather evidence on what tools work, and practical methods for applying them in routine settings. Other areas for research include how to reach out to communities, and how to provide training so that staff can become more involved and engaged in working with patients with similar cultural backgrounds. Throughout all of these efforts, there needs to be a focus on activities that reduce costs and have the most impact on population health.

PHARMACY PRACTICE

Gerald McEvoy, Pharm.D.
American Society of Health-Systems Pharmacists

Most patients leave a physician's office with a medication as part of an overall therapy regimen. Effective communication about medications is a key component of effective and safe use of therapy by patients, and is a core competency that will be required of pharmacists as they engage patients more directly in terms of care management. The information that patients encounter ranges from the label on the prescription container, to risk-benefit information, to participating in the decision with their physician as to whether or not they even want to receive a particular treatment. Patients must understand why it is that they are receiving a medicine, and why it is important to their overall health that they take it properly and regularly.

The American Society of Health-System Pharmacists (ASHP) represents pharmacists practicing in hospitals and organized health systems (e.g., acute care, ambulatory care clinics, hospital outpatient pharmacies, home care, long-term care). Pharmacists play a key role in managing medication therapy and reducing preventable harm.

The ACA and Pharmacy

The ASHP has, for many decades, fostered best practices that deal with quality issues for patient care, as well as the provision of information to patients. Historically, providing that information has been a core professional responsibility of pharmacists. Up to this point, much of those efforts involved communicating with other health care professionals, such as providing information to physicians to help them make a decision about a drug. Moving forward under the ACA, a key responsibility of pharmacists will be communicating effectively with patients to help them manage their health care with the medications that they have been prescribed. In this regard, there are a variety of tools that are available to help pharmacies assess their health literacy and training tools.

Disease prevention is another area in which pharmacists have established effective practices, covering areas such as diabetes, hypertension, cardiovascular disease, and tobacco cessation. Patient-centeredness is clearly an element of medication counseling, medication therapy management, and the U.S. Pharmacopeia (USP) prescription container labeling standards. As the key profession with expertise in medication therapy, pharmacists are integral to the collaborative-practice model that is at the core of medical homes. With regard to cultural competency and equity, there are a number of standards that apply to pharmacies (e.g., ASHP best practice on disparities in health care, Pharm.D. accreditation standards, ASHP residency standards).

Coverage expansion under the ACA will result in increased drug benefit coverage. Pharmacy workforce development is not addressed specifically in the ACA, and McEvoy said that the ASPH will be advocating for the need to include pharmacists as a profession in workforce development programs. With regard to patient information, the FDA is expected to issue new standards for the provision of written information to patients in 2012.

McEvoy highlighted several sections of the ACA that are key areas for pharmacy stakeholders (Box 4-1). Section 3503, addressing medication therapy management services, is the cornerstone of the ACA in terms of pharmacy practice, he said. The goal is to optimize medication use for improved patient outcomes, and to improve communication between patients and the health care team regarding their therapeutic regimen. Section 3507 addresses patient information on risks and benefits, which is most useful when provided at the point of prescribing as opposed to the point of dispensing.

Collaborative Opportunities with Pharmacy

Communication is at the core of all of the opportunities for pharmacies under health care reform. Communicating benefits and risks to both patients and prescribers to facilitate informed decisions about therapy is paramount.

There are special medication risk management issues for the elderly, including concerns about health literacy; polypharmacy and simplifying regimens; adjusted dosing and explaining to patients the importance of taking the prescribed dosage and not altering it on their own; and the use of drugs that may contribute to risks that the elderly face (such as falls). Adherence to drug therapy, risk evaluation and mitigation strategies for high-risk drugs, and medication therapy management are other areas where there are opportunities for pharmacy.

With regard to the patient-centered medical home, most medications require assessment of effectiveness. About one-third of all adverse effects leading to hospitalization are attributable to medication. Only about 30 to 50 percent of patients with chronic conditions adhere to their prescribed medication therapies, and medication cost is an important cause of low adherence. Pharmacists can play an important role in managing therapies by reviewing the therapy that the patient is receiving; identifying cost-effective therapies and optimizing outcomes; resolving medication-related problems; optimizing complex regimens; designing and managing adherence programs; and finally, educating patients about the safe and effective use of their medications.

BOX 4-1
Key ACA Provisions for Pharmacy Stakeholders

- Sec. 3503 Medication therapy management (MTM) services
  - o Focus on patient-centered rather than product-centered process of care
  - o Optimize medication use for improved patient outcomes
  - o Improve communication between patients and the healthcare team

- Sec. 3507 Prescription drug benefit and risk information
  - o Present patient with benefit-risk information at point of prescribing (i.e., decision point); too late at dispensing point

- Sec. 10328 improve Part D MTM programs
  - o Support access to MTM by all Medicare Part D beneficiaries

- Sec. 6301 Patient-centered outcomes research
  - o Submitted nominations to the Patient Centered Outcomes Research Institute
  - o Pharmacy members of AHRQ's pharmacy stakeholder advisory committee will recommend comparative effectiveness research and other activities

- Sec. 5307 Cultural competency, prevention, and public health
  - o Included in education, residency training, and professional practice standards

- Sec. 3021 Center for Medicare and Medicaid Innovation
  - o Advocate adoption of elements of MTM as part of development and testing of new care models

- Sec. 5305 Geriatric education and training

- Chronic disease testing and treatment, medication reconciliation, cognitive impairment assessment, and wellness guidance for elderly

- Meaningful use of electronic health records

- Patient-centered care models such as medical home
  - o Pharmacist collaboration for medication therapy services

---

SOURCE: McEvoy, 2010

Health literacy opportunities include effective communication through the prescription container label, comprehensible patient-centered supplemental materials, and clear counseling, education, and training. One of the elements in the ACA, for example, is testing of a "drug facts box" that came out of research at Dartmouth about patient understanding of risk-benefit information.

Challenges

Among the principal challenges moving forward is the fact that medication therapy is becoming increasingly complex. The more complex therapy becomes, the more difficult it is to explain to the patient the importance of how to take the medication properly, any associated risks with that medication, and what the potential benefits to them as a patient might be. Medications are also becoming increasingly specialized and individualized, pushing the limits of the expertise of the health care professional to effectively explain the therapy. The cost of medications is also increasing. In addition to the communication challenges related to the therapies themselves, the consumer population is aging and becoming increasingly more diverse.

Pharmacy is currently engaged in addressing these challenges. The ASHP Pharmacy Practice Model Initiative, for example, is focused on direct patient care as opposed to delivery of product. The Center for Health Transformation's 21st Century Intelligent Pharmacy Project is conducting similar pilot work looking at the transformation of pharmacy practice as a key component in providing affordable health care. Other projects are focused on specific diseases, such as the Asheville Project, where pharmacists managed four diseases for the city of Asheville, North Carolina, and the Diabetes Ten City Challenge.

These various programs and pilot projects show how pharmacist involvement in managing therapy with patients can be highly cost-effective, and highly effective in terms of patient outcomes in managing their disease.

DISCUSSION

Eligibility

A participant shared a hypothetical example of how people who qualify for Medicaid are not necessarily a steady population. Based on changing personal health, employment, and financial circumstances, they can migrate from Medicaid to the health insurance exchange to subsidized coverage by the federal government, and back again. Many are immigrants who have limited English-speaking capability and will be even more challenged to understand when they are eligible to be covered under what program. Funderburk recommended referring people to HealthCare.gov as a starting place, although currently the available languages are limited to English and Spanish. CMS is developing the health insurance portal such that it will ask individuals questions about their current situation and then show them the options that are available to them, allowing them to contrast and compare those options.

Another factor that comes into play for patients on the cusp of eligibility is whether they are being treated for an acute or chronic condition, McEvoy added. A patient with a chronic condition would, it is hoped, be in a managed setting or be engaged in medication therapy management, and would have an advocate, an established, trusted relationship with a provider or practice who can help him or her navigate the coverage process.

Scholle said that under the new standards for medical homes, practices are expected to be asking these kinds of questions and helping patients to determine what coverage they are eligible for. Even better would be a practice that is connected to a community center that can help with language and cultural needs.

Choosing Quality Care

An important market driver of quality is consumer demand. But when considering health care, most people do not know what quality is and as a result, there is no consumer demand for quality health care. Health literacy can help make quality more understandable to consumers. Scholle noted that the NCQA conducted focus groups of people who are treated in medical home practices and others from the same community who are in other practices. People in the medical home model were very happy with their care and understood and appreciated the concept of coordinated care, while the other group was skeptical of the whole idea (although neither was familiar with the term *medical home*). This supports the idea that there is no consumer demand because consumers often do not know what to demand until they have experienced it. We need to get people to think that managing their health is important, and give them experience with quality health systems that support that care, she said. The choice architecture concept supports this as well, by building decision frameworks that make it easy for people to choose what is good for them, even though they might not understand all of the elements.

Funderburk concurred that choice architecture is critical. The term *medical home* leads some to believe that they are losing control over their care. Better coordination could be achieved by being transparent and building on existing trusted relationships (e.g., a primary provider gives out his email or mail address and says, "If you go to another doctor, let me know because I think we could work together and make your care better for you"). The patient does not have to be an activated consumer, he or she just has to think that it sounds like a good idea.

Strategies and Interventions

Participants discussed further the concept of a multistakeholder coordinated strategy raised by Pisano. A coordinated effort gives the issue a louder voice, Pisano said. Such a strategy would likely involve some elements of the regulatory process, as well as involvement of consumer organizations. Consumer research would be needed to determine where to focus to achieve the greatest impact, and what should be the priorities. It is not possible to design major programs around every element of the ACA, she noted.

While accountable care organizations are potentially the best way of implementing health literacy practices, the incentives for establishment of ACOs are not yet clearly defined. Scholle said that the goal is to define a care structure that will incentivize provider organizations to work together to achieve the best results for the population with regard to health, reduced costs, and improved patient experiences. This involves motivating patients to become involved in improving their health and avoiding the need for hospitalization. The incentives will likely be financial, and there are opportunities to be involved in helping to define them as various agencies (e.g., the NCQA, CMS) are currently developing standards and calling for comments.

A question was raised about what actually constitutes a health literacy intervention. A participant said that when AHRQ conducted a review of the literature in 2004, they defined a health literacy intervention study as one that assessed the impact of an intervention on those with known limited health literacy. In other words, studies that measured the impact of a program on the overall population were not included, as they could actually be increasing disparities (people with higher health literacy reap most of the benefit while those with lower health literacy are left behind). This is a relatively narrow definition, and there are many relevant interventions that would not necessarily be called health literacy interventions.

Advice for Implementers

A participant asked panelists what their advice would be to those that are now charged with implementing the ACA, in terms of inserting health literacy into program design now, as opposed to having to retrofit it later. Scholle noted that there is no requirement for the reading level of informational materials in the medical home standards, in part because of the burden it would place on small physician practices. There needs to be an easy way to provide plain language materials at the appropriate reading level to practices. Second, workforce training is not just for physicians. A workforce strategy needs to encompass all health care providers and staff. Funderburk said that providers also need well-designed, simple, step-by-step information and systems so they are not wasting their limited time trying to figure out how to be in compliance. Pisano added that it is critical to engage patients in the implementation process.

5

How Can Health Literacy
Facilitate Health Care Reform?

George Isham, M.D.
HealthPartners

It is clear from the workshop discussions that the ACA touches everything we do, Isham said. As written, health literacy is not a primary principle of the new law, and the challenge of incorporating health literacy into mainstream American health care persists. This new legislation will dominate the political debate for some time to come, and implementation will span at least the next decade. In addition to the ACA, there were three other major health policy initiatives in 2010: the National Action Plan to Improve Health Literacy; the Plain Writing Act of 2010; and the launch of *Healthy People 2020*. We must continue to keep health literacy relevant to these processes, Isham said.

The ongoing political debate creates a barrier to helping people understand how provisions of the ACA may help them with their health care. There are competing messages about the reforms, stemming from advertising and positioning statements from both the political left and right. The information the public is getting may not bear any relationship to the reality of the legislation. We need to help people better understand this information so they can act on their own behalf for their own health.

The ACA sets new expectations for consumers. Health decisions will need to be made by people with all levels of health literacy. Isham raised several questions for consideration: how will consumers be touched by the tools and initiatives that are already in place; what fraction will be influenced by government websites, television, advertising of one type or another, or by friends and neighbors, and will the information they obtain be accurate or appropriate? We need to better understand the ecology of health decision making and how to achieve the greatest impact at the population level. Toolkits, websites, and projects are good starts, Isham said, but they are only the very firsts step in a chain of implementations.

Another question is how to measure the success of the ACA. Metrics could relate to process, financial gain or loss, or health outcomes. A related question is how to dissect out the impact of health literacy initiatives.

Throughout the workshop there was discussion about the relationship between quality improvement and health literacy. Researchers may want to study the impacts of quality and literacy in isolation. A practical implementer, however, will need to address these factors together, and in concert with other elements to achieve the desired impact.

Prioritizing will be important. There is much to be done, and areas of focus will need to be identified. We must start by understanding what people need to be well, and what they need to get better when they are ill. Isham supported the idea of segmenting by market, in other words, identifying the needs of seniors, children, and other vulnerable or underserved populations. Once we understand what they need, the next questions are what, objectively, is the status of current efforts on those issues, and what should be the short- and long-term goals going forward? The next questions that would follow are, what measures exist to be able to assess implementation for quality improvement and accountability, and what resources are available to be able to take action? It will then be important to continually cycle back to look at customer needs.

Isham identified Medicaid expansion as the primary opportunity to impact health literacy. Two targets in the implementation are the exchanges and choice. Health literacy will be a factor for underserved populations in these areas.

There are concerns about changes to the delivery system, and we need to think in terms of how health literacy is embedded in health system transformation. With accountable care organizations, for example, how will shared savings be spent? Will they be returned to the accountable care organizations since they created them? Will they be returned to consumers in the form of lower premiums? Will they be reinvested to address other issues? Another charge for accountable care organizations is to know their populations and be able to measure the health literacy of those they serve.

Isham also highlighted the workshop discussions regarding the importance of making the business case for health literacy. Success will involve cultural change, management change, leadership, and innovation.

And there must be better connection and cooperation across all political subdivisions (federal, state, and community).

Ruth Parker, M.D.
Emory University School of Medicine

Health literacy is fundamental to health care reform. It is the foundation upon which efforts to reduce disparities, reduce costs, and improve quality can be built. We need to find ways to make health literacy a priority on the front-end, Parker said, rather than as an afterthought. Voluntary guidance and good will are not likely to be sufficient, and some level of oversight and enforcement will be needed to ensure that health literacy is addressed. The challenge is how to do this, as it is not written into the law.

Parker supported the concept of choice architecture that makes it easier for patients to make good choices. She highlighted enrollment and medication labels as areas where there are prime opportunities for action on health literacy now, as well as the Center for Medicare and Medicaid Innovation funding ideas that are specific to health literacy. There are also opportunities for synergy of ACA-related efforts with the Plain Language Act.

Medicine at its simplest is supposed to be about people and their health. Yet providers often end up in silos of their expertise. Providers need to come together and put greater value on the health of the public and the health of patients.

Scott Ratzan, M.D.
Johnson & Johnson

Ratzan expressed concern that while health literacy is at the tipping point, there is a lack of leadership or ownership of the issue, and a lack of enthusiasm for finding the answers. There is a solid evidence base for health literacy. The task now is to take the disparate parts of health reform that are law, and that have some funding, and put together a national action plan or health literacy campaign that links across the different agency areas and efforts.

The roundtable can contribute by bringing people from outside fields into the health conversation. Specifically, Ratzan recommended looking to fields such as behavioral economics to learn more about how people make choices. Choices are affected by how something is presented, as well as by misunderstandings. Ratzen noted that he has heard insurers say that communication campaigns do not work and that the focus should be on service delivery. This is not the case, and there is a strong evidence base for communications in other fields that can be drawn upon.

Government action alone may not be sufficient and public-private partnerships will likely play a role. We need to have strong leadership that will harness the available technology and help develop a campaign of knowledge and skills to reach the public and the learned intermediaries, the pharmacists, nurses, physicians, physical therapists, and front-line health workers.

GENERAL DISCUSSION

Many participants agreed with Ratzan that there is a critical need for leadership on this issue. There has been tremendous progress in terms of a number of organizations that originally seemed unlikely to embrace health literacy, and within different work groups in the government, and there are some health literacy champions within government. But while there is much talk about health literacy being at the tipping point, as of yet there is no valid commitment to begin to implement health literacy in a meaningful way. A participant suggested that some people are waiting to see if health literacy will "go away" and if there will be other priorities and funding streams that will take precedence. Health literacy must be embraced and implemented in programs the participant said. In this regard, leadership, both public and private, needs to make a statement of commitment.

Another participant suggested that some of the expectations around this legislation are somewhat unrealistic. The ACA will help coverage expansion, he said, but it is only a first step toward health reform. Health literacy can and should be the guiding light for that forthcoming reform. It was also noted that the ACA is focused on health care coverage issues as opposed to health issues. Health literacy has as much to do with health promotion and wellness as it does with the health care delivery system.

A participant from a leading health care organization said that they are working to accurately depict what the choices are for what is really a new membership group under health care reform, a generation of individuals who have never had health insurance. It is not just about enrolling them, but about giving them a patient experience and a health care delivery system that meets their needs. Health literacy is not separate, but will be manifested in how we do in terms of meeting their expectations and reaching the desired clinical outcomes.

Participants discussed the challenges of having so many different tools, developed by so many different organizations (e.g., diabetes fact sheets). It would be helpful and more resource-efficient if there were better coordination in developing standardized, easy to use, and easy to obtain materials.

It was also noted that to really make a difference in health literacy, it is important to engage at a community level. States also need to have the opportunity to develop approaches that best reflect their population's needs.

A participant raised a specific concern that under Section 2953 of the ACA (Personal Responsibility Education), funding is restricted to education of young adults on reproductive health (pregnancy prevention, sexually transmitted diseases). Health is a lifelong responsibility, he emphasized.

In closing the discussion, Ratzan said that with regard to an evidence-based approach to health communications, we know where people get their information. There are ways to reach them by television, radio, friends, mobile phone, digital device, and new technologies. Now is the time to take action and reach out to them. Parker added that throughout the day it was repeated that people do not understand what the ACA is about, and what it means for them individually. She suggested an accessible, actionable guide to the ACA, addressing the three target populations that were discussed, vulnerable individuals, children, and senior citizens with health concerns, would be a valuable document.

References

Advisory Commission on Consumer Protection and Quality in the Health Care Industry. 1998. *Quality first: better health care for all Americans: final report to the President of the United States*. Washington, DC: Government Printing Office.

AHRQ (Agency for Healthcare Research and Quality). 2010. *Health literacy universal precautions toolkit*. http://www.ahrq.gov/qual/literacy/ (accessed February 24, 2011).

Berkman, N. D., D. A. Dewalt, M. P. Pignone, S. L. Sheridan, K. N. Lohr, L. Lux, S. F. Sutton, T. Swinson, and A. J. Bonito. 2004. Literacy and health outcomes. *Evidence Report/Technology Assessment* (87):1-8.

Funderburk, F. 2010. Centers for Medicare and Medicaid Services. PowerPoint Presentation at the Institute of Medicine workshop on health literacy and healthcare reform. Washington, DC: Novermber 10.

HHS (Department of Health and Human Services). 2010. *National action plan to improve health literacy*. Washington, DC: Office of Disease Prevention and Health Promotion.

HHS. 2011. *Healthfinder.gov*. http://www.healthfinder.gov/ (accessed February 24, 2011).

Hibbard, J. H. 2009. Using systematic measurement to target consumer activation strategies. *Medical Care Research and Review* 66(Suppl 1):9S-27S.

Holahan, J., A. Cook, and L. Dubay. 2007. *Characteristics of the uninsured: who is eligible for public coverage and who needs help affording coverage?* Washington, DC: Kaiser Family Foundation, Commission on Medicaid and the Uninsured. http://www.kff.org/uninsured/upload/7613.pdf (accessed February 24, 2011).

IOM (Institute of Medicine). 2004. *Health literacy: a prescription to end confusion*. Washington, DC: The National Academies Press.

McEvoy, G. 2010. Pharmacy Practice. PowerPoint Presentation at the Institute of Medicine workshop on health literacy and health care reform. Washington, DC: November 10.

Perrin, J. M. 2002. Health services research for children with disabilities. *Milbank Quarterly* 80(2):303-324.

Sanders, L. M., S. Federico, M. Abrams, B. Dreyer, W. Cull, J. Ohone-Frempong, and T. Davis. 2007. Readability of enrollment forms for the State Children's Health Insurance Program (SCHIP). In *Pediatric Academic Societies Meeting, American Academy of Pediatrics Presidential Plenary*. Toronto, Canada.

Sanders, L. M. 2010 Children. PowerPoint Presentation at the Institute of Medicine workshop on health literacy and healthcare reform. Washington, DC: Novermber 10.

Turner, T., W. L. Cull, B. Bayldon, P. Klass, L. M. Sanders, M. Frintner, M. Abrams, and B. Dreyer. 2009. Pediatricians and health literacy: descriptive results from a national survey. *Pediatrics* 124(Suppl 3):S299-S305.

Yin, H. S., B. P. Dreyer, G. Foltin, L. van Schaick, and A. L. Mendelsohn. 2007. Association of low caregiver health literacy with reported use of nonstandardized dosing instruments and lack of knowledge of weight-based dosing. *Ambulatory Pediatrics* 7(4):292-298.

Yin, H. S., B. P. Dreyer, L. van Schaick, G. L. Foltin, C. Dinglas, and A. L. Mendelsohn. 2008. Randomized controlled trial of a pictogram-based intervention to reduce liquid medication dosing errors and improve adherence among caregivers of young children. *Archives of Pediatrics and Adolescent Medicine* 162(9):814-822.

Yin, H. S., A. L. Mendelsohn, M. S. Wolf, R. M. Parker, A. Fierman, L. van Schaick, I. S. Bazan, M. D. Kline, and B. P. Dreyer. 2010. Parents' medication administration errors: role of dosing instruments and health literacy. *Archives of Pediatrics and Adolescent Medicine* 164(2):181-186.

A

Workshop Agenda

8:30-8:45   Welcome and Introduction
              George Isham, M.D., M.S.
              Chair, IOM Roundtable on Health Literacy

8:45-9:15   Health Literacy and the Patient Protection and Affordable
              Care Act
              Stephen Somers, Ph.D.   *Roopa Mahadevan, M.A.*
              President   *Program Associate*
              Center for Health Care   *Center for Health Care*
              Strategies   *Strategies*

9:15-9:30   2010—The Year of Health Literacy
              Anand Parekh, M.D., M.P.H.
              Deputy Assistant Secretary for Health

9:30-10:15   Discussion

10:15-10:30   BREAK

**10:30-12:15   PANEL: Opportunities for and Challenges to Individuals
              Under the New Law**

Participants will be sent the commissioned paper in advance. Speaking
within the context of the paper, each will be asked to identify the health
literacy opportunities and challenges to *individuals* within the provisions
of the law.

10:30-10:45   Vulnerable Populations
              Cheryl Bettigole, M.D.
              Clinical Director, HC#10
              Philadelphia Department of Health

10:45-11:00   Children
              Lee Sanders, M.D., M.P.H.
              Associate Professor
              University of Miami
              Miller School of Medicine

11:00-11:15   Seniors with Health Problems
              Harold Fallon, M.D.
              Dean Emeritus
              School of Medicine
              University of Alabama at Birmingham

11:15-11:30   Populations with Behavioral Health Issues*
              Carolyn Cocotas, R.T., M.P.A.
              Senior Vice President
              Quality and Corporate Compliance
              F.E.G.S. Health and Human Services System

11:30-12:15   Discussion

12:15-1:15   LUNCH

**1:15-3:00   PANEL: Opportunities for and Challenges to Those
                     Implementing the Law**

Participants will be sent the commissioned paper in advance. Speaking
within the context of the paper, each will be asked to identify the
health literacy opportunities and challenges to *organizations* involved in
implementing the provisions of the law.

              1:15-1:30   CMS
                          Frank Funderburk
                          Director, Division of Research
                          Center for Medicare and Medicaid Services

---

* Carolyn Cocotas was unable to attend the workshop.

1:30-1:45 Insurer
Susan Pisano, M.A.
Vice President of Communications
America's Health Insurance Plans

1:45-2:00 Quality
Sarah Scholle, Dr.P.H.
Assistant Vice President for Research and
Analysis
National Committee on Quality Assurance

2:00-2:15 American Society of Health System Pharmacists
Gerald McEvoy, Pharm.D.
Assistant Vice President for Drug Information
American Society of Health-Systems Pharmacists

2:15-3:00 Discussion

3:00-3:30 PANEL: How Can Health Literacy Facilitate Health Care Reform?

Each speaker will have 10 minutes to describe what he or she identifies as ways in which health literacy can facilitate the implementation of provisions in the Patient Protection and Affordable Care Act
George Isham, M.D., Medical Director and Chief Health Officer
HealthPartners
Ruth Parker, M.D., Professor of Medicine
Emory University School of Medicine
Scott Ratzan, M.D., Vice President, Global Health
Johnson & Johnson

3:30-4:00 General Discussion

4:00 ADJOURN

B

Workshop Speaker Biosketches

Cheryl Bettigole, M.D., M.P.H., is a board certified family physician and the clinical director of a primary care clinic run by the Philadelphia Department of Public Health. In her work for the health department, she has cared for diverse populations of patients at city clinics since completing her residency in 1999. As clinical director, she has worked to improve services for patients of limited English proficiency and to implement a chronic disease management program. Dr. Bettigole is a member of the Health Reform Task Force of the Association of Clinicians for the Underserved and is the President-Elect of the National Physicians Alliance as well as a member of the American Academy of Family Physicians. She is a magna cum laude graduate of Jefferson Medical College, completed her residency in Family Medicine at Thomas Jefferson University Hospital, and completed her master's in Public Health at Johns Hopkins Bloomberg School of Public Health, where she received a Capstone award for her work on interpretation services in a public health clinic setting.

Carolyn Cocotas, R.T., M.P.A., is senior vice president of Quality and Corporate Compliance at F.E.G.S. Health and Human Services System, one of the largest voluntary, not-for-profit health, education, and human services organizations in the country. Previously, she was director of Community Health Innovation at Affinity Health Plan where she directed innovation work in care delivery to the Medicaid population. Ms. Cocotas' career spans over three decades during which she has held progressively responsible positions in the health care industry, including HHS,

U.S. Government Accountability Office, U.S. House of Representatives, National Committee for Quality Assurance, Community Health Plan of the Rockies, Performance Measurement Coordinating Council, and Kaiser Permanente. Ms. Cocotas has a master's degree in public and health administration from the University of New Mexico.

Harold Fallon, M.D., is a graduate of Yale College and Yale Medical School. His residency training in internal medicine was at UNC. He had further training at the National Cancer Institute and fellowships in liver disease at Yale and biochemistry at Duke. During 15 years on the faculty at UNC he developed a new liver disease program and directed research in liver lipid metabolism. He was Chair of the Department of Medicine at MCV (now VCU) in Richmond for 18 years and was then Dean of the University of Alabama School of Medicine in Birmingham. During his academic career he was Chair or President of numerous national medical and research organizations including the Board of Internal Medicine, the Association of American Physicians, the Association of Professors of Medicine, and the American College of Physicians. He was the first Home Secretary of the IOM and was Chairman of the series of annual Conferences on Health Literacy, jointly sponsored by the American College of Physicians Foundation (ACPF) and the IOM. He is retired, but remains active with various activities at the IOM, ACPF, and the Medical University of South Carolina.

Frank Funderburk joined the Division of Research in 2007. He is currently responsible for the strategic planning, implementation, and analysis of a variety of health care research efforts that support and enhance CMS communications activities. He is especially interested in developing data-driven communication strategies that can overcome persistent informational, attitudinal, and motivational barriers to better health care, including those related to health and digital literacy. His research has included evaluation of the effectiveness of a variety of outreach and education campaigns as well as a recent experimental study of direct marketing strategies for improving outreach to vulnerable beneficiaries eligible for but not enrolled in the Low Income Subsidy. He has investigated ways in which health care decision making style can influence beneficiary perception of Medicare programs as well as receptivity to specific outreach and communication activities. His work has helped to inform recent initiatives encouraging adoption of Electronic Health Records and quality initiatives such as the HCAHPS public reporting of consumers' hospital experiences.

Prior to joining CMS Frank was an Analytic Scientist at the Delmarva Foundation for Medical Care where he directed External Quality Review for Medicaid programs in 9 states and the District of Columbia. He also worked with states to develop innovative outreach programs to improve the quality of care and the quality of life of people receiving Medicaid.

Frank has over 20 years of health care, health communications, and health policy research experience ranging from basic scientific studies of brain-behavior relationships involved in decision-making to large multi-center clinical trials of new pharmaceutical products as well as national surveys of consumer behavior.

Roopa Mahadevan, M.A., is a Program Associate at the Center for Health Care Strategies (CHCS). Roopa works on CHCS programs aimed at improving the quality and cost-effectiveness of publicly-financed health care for children and youth through the Children in Managed Care (CIMC) initiative, Healthy Smiles—Healthy Families: Improving Oral Health for Children in California's Healthy Families Program project, and the CHIPRA Quality Demonstration Grant. Roopa also works on CHCS' racial/ethnic disparities portfolio, and is a member of its technical assistance team for the Robert Wood Johnson Foundation's Aligning Forces for Quality initiative. She additionally provides programmatic support to the Rethinking Care Program, a CHCS initiative focused on Medicaid's highest-need, complex adult populations.

Prior to joining CHCS, Roopa served as health care policy coordinator for Silicon Valley Leadership Group, working with Bay Area companies on issues of workplace wellness and health care reform. She has also been a part of research teams at the University of California, San Francisco, and Stanford University, investigating clinical and epidemiological issues related to chronic disease, mental health, and aging. After completing her graduate studies, she was awarded the U.S. Fulbright scholarship to pursue music performance training in India. While there, she participated in diabetes prevention research and community-based health literacy promotion activities for the Madras Diabetes Research Foundation, a WHO Collaborating Center for non-communicable disease.

Ms. Mahadevan received a master's degree in psychology/cognitive science and a bachelor's degree in biology, both from Stanford University.

Gerald K. McEvoy, Pharm.D., is assistant vice president of Drug Information at the American Society of Health-System Pharmacists (ASHP). In addition, Dr. McEvoy has served as editor-in-chief of AHFS Drug Information (AHFS DI), ASHP's federally recognized drug compendium, for over 28 years. In his capacities as AVP of Drug Information and Editor in Chief of AHFS DI and AHFS DI Consumer Medication information (AHFS DI CMI), Dr. McEvoy is responsible for a variety of publishing and database management projects within ASHP focusing on dissemination of drug information in both electronic and print formats to various audiences, including health professionals and patients. Through partnership with various health information vendors and other parties, including the National Library of Medicine, Consumer Reports, and Medscape/ WebMD, ASHP's professional and patient drug information is available as both referential and integrated data in a wide variety of services and settings. Dr. McEvoy has spoken widely on evidence-based development of drug prescribing information as well as on patient safety, emergency preparedness, and media-neutral publishing and electronic data interchange through SGML and XML data structuring and document tagging.

Dr. McEvoy currently serves on the BMJ Group North American Advisory Board, National Council on Patient Information and Education Board, USP Safe Medication Use Expert Committee, and USP Providers Advisory Forum for Medicare Part D Model Guidelines. Dr. McEvoy also served on an Institute of Medicine Panel on Changing Prescription Medication Use Container Instructions to Improve Health Literacy and Medication Safety and subsequently was appointed Co-chair of USP's Health Literacy and Prescription Container Labeling Advisory Panel, which he continues to co-chair. In addition, Dr McEvoy is a recognized authority on consumer medication information, testifying before and advising the U.S. Food and Drug Administration (FDA) on medication safety communication issues involving consumers, advising the Consumer Reports on medication use issues, and speaking internationally on the provision of safe medication use information to consumers.

Before joining ASHP, Dr. McEvoy obtained both his baccalaureate and doctorate degrees in Pharmacy from Duquesne University in Pittsburgh, Pennsylvania, and completed a hospital residency at Mercy Hospital in Pittsburgh. He recently was awarded the Duquesne University Pharmacy Alumni Achievement Award.

Anand K. Parekh, M.D., M.P.H., is the Deputy Assistant Secretary for Health (Science and Medicine) in the Office of the Assistant Secretary for Health at the U.S. Department of Health and Human Services. In this capacity, he provides oversight, direction, and coordination of activities pertaining to (1) a range of emerging public health and science issues; (2) the continuum of medical research—including clinical science and health services research; and (3) issues requiring expert medical analysis and advice, particularly those concerning policy, planning, formulation, and presentation of public health issues affecting the Department. Dr. Parekh has worked on a variety of health issues including public health emergency preparedness, pandemic and seasonal influenza preparedness, quality of care improvement, chronic care management, childhood obesity, HIV/AIDS, Lyme disease, and chronic fatigue syndrome. He also chairs the Department's Medical Claims Review Panel.

Dr. Parekh completed his undergraduate studies in political science as well as his graduate school training in medicine and public health at the University of Michigan. He subsequently completed his residency training in the Osler Medical Training Program of the Department of Medicine at Johns Hopkins Hospital. In addition to engaging in health services research at Johns Hopkins, Dr. Parekh has completed separate stints as a research fellow at the Centers for Medicare & Medicaid Services and at the Institute of Medicine.

Dr. Parekh maintains a Medical Staff position at Holy Cross Hospital in Silver Spring, Maryland, and practices at the Holy Cross Health Center—a low-cost adult medicine clinic for the uninsured. He is an Adjunct Assistant Professor in the Department of Medicine at Johns Hopkins Hospital. He also serves on the Board of Governors of the University of Michigan School of Public Health Alumni Society and is a member of the Presidential Scholars Alumni Society and the American College of Physicians.

Susan Pisano is the Vice President of Communications for America's Health Insurance Plans (AHIP). AHIP is a national association whose member companies provide health insurance coverage to more than 200 million Americans. The AHIP member companies offer medical insurance, long-term care insurance, disability income insurance, dental insurance, supplemental insurance, stop-loss insurance, and reinsurance to consumers, employers, and public purchasers. As Vice President for Communications, Susan acts as a spokesperson for AHIP and is responsible for outreach to member companies, the news media, and other major audiences. She is the primary staffer for AHIP's Health Literacy Task Force. Ms. Pisano has worked at AHIP since 1987. Before coming to AHIP she was the public relations director at Pacific Medical Center in Seattle, Washington, a local institution that had an HMO affiliated with it since 1985. Susan began her career at Pennsylvania Hospital in Philadelphia, where she attended Chestnut Hill College (B.A., 1971) and Villanova University (M.A., 1975).

Lee Sanders, M.D., M.P.H., is a general pediatrician and Associate Professor of Pediatrics at the University of Miami, Miller School of Medicine. A graduate of Harvard College, he completed medical school and pediatric residency at Stanford University and a research fellowship in public health at UCSF and UC Berkeley.

Dr. Sanders' clinical expertise is in the comprehensive care of children from birth through age 21. His clinical interests include the care complex chronic conditions, child development, and obesity prevention.

An author of numerous peer-reviewed articles and book chapters, Dr.

Sanders is a nationally recognized scholar in the field of health literacy. Dr. Sanders was named a Robert Wood Johnson Foundation Generalist Physician Faculty Scholar for his leadership on the role of health literacy in addressing child health disparities. Dr. Sanders' current research includes an NIH-funded study to assess the efficacy of a low-literacy, early-childhood intervention designed to prevent obesity, as well as locally funded efforts to improve health promotion through child-care centers, WIC offices, and farmers' markets.

Dr. Sanders currently serves as Medical Director of Children's Medical Services South Florida, a Florida state agency that coordinates care for more than 10,000 low-income children with special health care needs. He is also Medical Director for Reach Out and Read Florida, a pediatric-clinic-based program that provides books and early-literacy promotion to more than 200,000 underserved children. At the University of Miami, Dr. Sanders directs the Medical Student Pathway in Social Medicine, sponsored by Jay Weiss Center for Social Medicine and Health Equity, which trains students and residents in community-based participatory research.

Sarah Hudson Scholle, M.P.H, Dr.P.H., is a health services researcher and has responsibility for overseeing the development and implementation of NCQA's research agenda. Her research interests focus on assessing quality of health care and understanding consumer perceptions and preferences in health care, particularly for women and families. Dr. Scholle leads efforts to develop new approaches to quality measurement and evaluation of health care, including comprehensive well care for children and women, care coordination for vulnerable populations, and patient experiences with the medical home. Dr. Scholle's prior work supported the development of NCQA's recognition program for patient-centered medical homes and distinction programs for multicultural health care populations, as well as numerous quality measures.

Prior to joining NCQA, Dr. Scholle previously served as Associate Professor at the University of Pittsburgh School of Medicine. Dr. Scholle has numerous publications in major health services and women's health journals. She chairs a Health Services Research Merit Review Board for the Veterans Administration Health Services Research and Development Program. She also reviews manuscripts for a variety of journals (including *Health Services Research* and *Women's Health Issues*). She has served on expert panels for the Institute of Medicine and the National Quality Forum. Dr. Scholle received her bachelor's degree in history and master's degree in public health from Yale University and her doctorate in public health from the Johns Hopkins University School of Hygiene and Public Health.

Stephen A. Somers, Ph.D., is the president and chief executive officer of the Center for Health Care Strategies (CHCS), which he founded in 1995 with a major grant on Medicaid-managed care from the Robert Wood Johnson Foundation. In that role, he is responsible for the organization's growth into a nationally recognized center on improving care for beneficiaries of this country's publicly financed health care programs, particularly those with chronic illnesses and disabilities and those experiencing racial and ethnic disparities in care. CHCS now receives support from multiple philanthropies, corporate community benefit programs, and the federal government.

Before starting CHCS, Dr. Somers was an associate vice president and program officer at the Robert Wood Johnson Foundation. Prior to that, he was a professional staff member at the U.S. Senate Special Committee on Aging and legislative assistant to U.S. Senator John Heinz of Pennsylvania. Dr. Somers serves as a visiting lecturer at Princeton University's Woodrow Wilson School of Public and International Affairs. Dr. Somers earned his Ph.D. in the politics of education from Stanford University.

C

CHCS

Center for
Health Care Strategies, Inc.

Health Literacy
Implications of the
Affordable Care Act

Commissioned by:
The Institute of Medicine

Authored by:
Stephen A. Somers, PhD
Roopa Mahadevan, MA

Center for Health Care Strategies, Inc.

69

Contents

The Center for Health Care Strategies (CHCS) is a nonprofit health policy resource center dedicated to improving health care quality for low-income children and adults, people with chronic illnesses and disabilities, frail elders, and racially and ethnically diverse populations experiencing disparities in care. CHCS works with state and federal agencies, health plans, providers and consumer groups to develop innovative programs that better serve Medicaid beneficiaries with complex and high-cost health care needs. Its program priorities are: improving quality and reducing racial and ethnic disparities; integrating care for people with complex and special needs; and building Medicaid leadership and capacity.

Acknowledgements

The authors thank Sara Rosenbaum, Hirsh Professor and Chair of Health Policy at George Washington University, for her cogent analysis of the legislation and insights into the opportunities it presents for promoting health literacy. We also wish to acknowledge the contributions of our colleagues at CHCS, particularly Stacey Chazin, Michael Canonico, and Dorothy Lawrence, for their assistance in preparing this document.

I.   Health Literacy and Health Care Reform

A lthough low health literacy is certainly not a featured concern of the health care reform legislation passed in early 2010, there are those who would argue that the law cannot be successful without a redoubling of national efforts to address the issue. Nearly 36 percent of America's adult population — 87 million adults — have low health literacy.[1] As the Patient Protection and Affordable Care Act (ACA) extends health insurance coverage to some 32 million lower-income adults and promotes greater attention to the barriers faced by individual patients, those implementing the law should consider how to incorporate health literacy into strategies for enrolling beneficiaries and delivering care.

For the purposes of this paper, health literacy is defined, using the National Library of Medicine's definition, as: *"The degree to which individuals have the capacity to obtain, process, and understand basic health information and services needed to make appropriate health decisions."*[2]

Fortunately, several ACA provisions directly acknowledge the need for greater attention to health literacy, and many others imply it. The law includes provisions to communicate health and health care information clearly; promote prevention; be patient-centered and create medical or health homes; assure equity and cultural competence; and deliver high-quality care. This paper identifies both the direct and indirect links, and provides those concerned about health literacy with provision-specific opportunities to support advancements. These provisions fall into six health and health care domains in the legislation where further action may be called for by concerned stakeholders:

(1) **Coverage expansion**: enrolling, reaching out to, and delivering care to health insurance coverage expansion populations in 2014 and beyond;
(2) **Equity**: assuring equity in health and health care for all communities and populations;
(3) **Workforce**: training providers on cultural competency, language, and literacy issues
(4) **Patient information** at appropriate reading levels;
(5) **Public health and wellness**; and
(6) **Quality improvement**: innovation to create more effective and efficient models of care, particularly for those with chronic illnesses requiring extensive self-management.

Individuals with low levels of health literacy are least equipped to benefit from the ACA, with potentially costly consequences for both those who pay for and deliver their care, as well as for themselves. Rates of low literacy are disproportionately high among lower-income Americans eligible for publicly financed care through Medicare or Medicaid.[3] In 2014, this pattern is likely to extend to individuals newly eligible for Medicaid or for publicly subsidized private insurance through state-based exchanges.

---

[1] Vernon, J, Trujillo, A, Rosenbaum, S, DeBuono, B. *Low Health Literacy: Implications for National Health Policy.* University of Connecticut: 2007

[2] Ratzan and Parker. 2000. Introduction. In: *National Library of Medicine Current Bibliographies in Medicine: Health Literacy.* NLM Pub. No. CBM 2000-1

[3] Kutner, M. et al *The Health Litearcy of America's Adults: Results from the 2003 National Assessment of Adult Literacy.* Washington, DC: U.S.Department of Education, National Center for Education, 2006

Health Literacy Until Now

In its *Healthy People 2010* aims statement, the Department of Health and Human Services (HHS) adopted the definition from the National Library of Medicine, declaring health literacy to be an important national health priority. *Healthy People 2010* broadened this definition to note that health literacy is not just the problem of the individual, but also a by-product of system-level contributions.[4] Acknowledging the salience of this issue, HHS Secretary Kathleen Sebelius made official a federal commitment to health literacy by releasing in May 2010 the *National Action Plan to Improve Health Literacy*[5]. The plan lays out seven goals that emphasize the importance of creating health and safety information that is accurate, accessible and actionable. It addresses payers, the media, government agencies, health care professionals and others, recognizing the multi-sector effort that will be required to effectively tackle this oft-ignored, national problem.

The U.S. health care system, with its myriad public and private programs, institutions, services, products, and information, poses a significant challenge to those seeking access to affordable, quality health care. Understanding the complexities of insurance eligibility, therapeutic guidance, medical technology, prescription medication, disease management, prevention, and lifestyle modification are difficult for any consumer, let alone one with compromised levels of literacy or numeracy (or quantitative literacy). An individual seeking to participate successfully in the health system requires a constellation of skills — reading, writing, basic mathematical calculations, speaking, listening, networking, and rhetoric — the totality of which defines health literacy.

However, national data suggest that only 12 percent of adults have proficient health literacy.[6] While low health literacy is found across all demographic groups, it disproportionately affects non-white racial and ethnic groups; the elderly; individuals with lower socioeconomic status and education; people with physical and mental disabilities; those with low English proficiency (LEP); and non-native speakers of English[7]. Low health literacy is associated with reduced use of preventive services and management of chronic conditions, and higher mortality[8]. It also leads to medication errors, misdiagnosis due to poor communication between providers and patients, low rates of guidance and treatment compliance, hospital readmissions, unnecessary emergency room visits, longer hospital stays, fragmented access to care, and poor responsiveness to public health emergencies. Accordingly, low health literacy has been estimated to cost the U.S. economy between $106 billion and $236 billion annually.[9]

The consequences of low health literacy have been recognized by federal agencies such as the Agency for Healthcare Research and Quality (AHRQ), the Centers for Disease Control and Prevention (CDC), the Food and Drug Administration (FDA), the Office of the Surgeon General, and the National Institutes of Health (NIH), as well as by private organizations such as America's Health Insurance Plans, the American College of Physicians, the American Medical Association, The Joint Commission on Accreditation, Kaiser Permanente, and Pfizer. These entities and many

---

[4] Rudd R. Objective 11-2. Improvement of Health Literacy. In: *Communicating Health: Priorities and Strategies for Progress*. Washington, DC: Office of Diseae Prevention and Health Promotion, U.S. Department of Health and Human Services.

[5] U.S. Department of Health and Human Services, Office of Disease Prevention and Health Promotion. *National Action Plan to Improve Health Literacy*. Washington, DC. 2010

[6] 2003 National Assessment of Adult Literacy (NAAL), National Center for Education Statistics, U.S. Department of Education

[7] Neilsen-Bohlman, L. Panzer A.M, Kindig, D.A. *Health Literacy: A Prescription to End Confusion*. Washington DC, National Academies Press. 2004

[8] Berkman et al. *Literacy and Health Outcomes*. Agency for Healthcare Research and Quality (AHRQ). Rockville, MD: 2004

[9] Vernon, J, Trujillo, A, Rosenbaum, S, DeBuono, B. *Low Health Literacy: Implications for National Health Policy*. University of Connecticut: 2007

others are promoting awareness, creating program initiatives, funding targeted research, setting readability standards, working with e-health and social media platforms, and providing tools and resources for measurement and quality improvement across providers, health plans, hospitals, and employer organizations. Important policy papers such as the Institute of Medicine's (IOM) 2004 report, *Health Literacy: A Prescription to End Confusion,*[10] and national data such as those produced by the National Adult Literacy Survey[11] have contributed to the knowledge base for this issue.

To date, however, strong legislative language, regulations, and appropriations for concerted efforts to address health literacy have not emerged from the federal government. Congressional bills such as the National Health Literacy Act of 2007[12] and the Plain Language Act of 2009,[13] which mapped out meaningful health literacy strategies, have not yet made it to the President's desk. It remains to be seen whether the ACA can be used to push the national health literacy agenda forward.

II. Health Literacy and the Affordable Care Act

T he ACA is, by any measure, a major piece of domestic policy legislation, directly affecting tens of millions of Americans at a cost of nearly one trillion dollars over the next 10 years.

The law's primary goals are to increase access to coverage, regulate the private insurance industry to allow more Americans into the system at affordable rates, and begin to control the rate of growth in health care costs. These goals cannot be achieved, however, without efforts to address cultural, linguistic and social barriers to care facing vulnerable populations. Low health literacy is critical among these barriers. The following ACA provisions include direct and indirect language concerning health literacy:

Definition

Title V, Subtitle A (amending existing laws and creating new law related to the health care workforce) of ACA establishes a statutory definition of "health literacy" consistent with *Healthy People 2010.* The term is defined as "the degree to which an individual has the capacity to obtain, communicate, process, and understand health information and services in order to make appropriate health decisions." Other direct mentions of health literacy do not specifically cross-reference the Title V definition (though presumably, HHS will use this terminology when implementing the various titles of the law).

Direct Mentions

Table 1 contains the law's four other direct mentions of the term health literacy. These provisions touch on issues of research dissemination, shared decision-making, medication labeling, and workforce development. All four suggest the need to communicate effectively with consumers, patients, and communities in order to improve the access to and quality of health care. None of these provisions creates explicit health literacy programs, specifies implementation or regulatory

---

[10] Neilsen-Bohlman, L. Panzer A.M, Kindig, D.A. *Health Literacy: A Prescription to End Confusion.* Washington DC, National Academies Press. 2004

[11] 2003 National Assessment of Adult Literacy (NAAL), National Center for Education Statistics, U.S. Department of Education. Washington DC.2006

[12] US Congress. S. 2424: National Health Literacy Act of 2007. 110th Congress. 2007 – 2008. Accessible at http://www.govtrack.us/congress/bill.xpd?bill=s110-2424

[13] US Congress. H.R. 946: Plain Writing Act of 2010. 11th Congreass 2009 – 2010. Accessible at http://www.govtrack.us/congress/bill.xpd?bill=h111-946

supports, or expounds further on the term "health literacy" beyond its mention. However, they are all consistent with the themes of patient-centeredness and overall quality improvement that are found more broadly throughout the legislation.

ACA Provisions with Direct References to "Health Literacy"

Section Number	Provision Title	Legislative Language
Sec. 3501	Health Care Delivery System Research; Quality Improvement Technical Assistance	Requires that research of the AHRQ's Center for Quality Improvement and Patient Safety be made "available to the public through multiple media and appropriate formats to reflect the varying needs of health care providers and consumers and diverse levels of **health literacy**."
Sec. 3506	Program to Facilitate Shared Decision-making	Amends the Public Health Service Act to "facilitate collaborative processes between patients, caregivers, authorized representatives and clinicians that enables decision-making, provides information about tradeoffs among treatment options, and facilitates the incorporation of patient preferences and values into the medical plan."
		Authorizes a "program to update patient decision aids to assist health care providers and patients." The program, administered by the CDC and NIH, awards grants and contracts to develop, update, and produce patient decision aids for preference-sensitive care to assist providers in educating patients, caregivers, and authorized representatives concerning the relative safety, effectiveness and cost of treatment, or where appropriate, palliative care. "Decision aids must reflect varying needs of consumers and diverse levels of **health literacy**."
Sec. 3507	Presentation of Prescription Drug Benefit and Risk Information	Directs the Secretary to determine whether the addition of certain standardized information to prescription drug labeling and print advertising would improve health care decision-making by clinicians and patients and consumers; to consider scientific evidence on decision-making; and to consult with various stakeholders and "experts in **health literacy**."
Sec. 5301	Training in Family Medicine, General Internal Medicine, General Pediatrics, and Physician Assistantship	Amends Title VII of the Public Health Service Act to permit the Secretary to make training grants in the primary care medical specialties. Preference for awards are for qualified applicants that "provide training in enhanced communication with patients. . . and in cultural competence and **health literacy**."

Indirect Provisions

Other instances where the concept of health literacy could come into play include those discussed in the following sections, organized into the six domains introduced at the outset. See the appendices for an extensive list and descriptions of these and other provisions.

Insurance Reform, Outreach, and Enrollment

Insurance Reform, Outreach, and Enrollment *(e.g., of populations newly eligible for Medicaid or insurance premium subsidies)*	
Section Number	**Provision Title**
Sec. 1002	Health Insurance Consumer Information
Sec. 1103	Immediate Information that Allows Consumers to Identify Affordable Coverage Options
Sec. 1311.	Affordable Choices of Health Benefit Plans *(includes language on "culturally and linguistically appropriate" obligations for plans)*
Sec. 1413	Streamlining of procedures for enrollment through an Exchange and State Medicaid, CHIP, and health subsidy programs
Sec. 2715.	Development and utilization of uniform explanation of coverage documents and standardized definitions.
Sec. 3306.	Funding outreach and assistance for low-income programs.

Health insurance market reforms have substantial potential for reducing inequities in the health system that are interrelated with insurance status. For example, the National Assessment of Adult Literacy found that adults with no insurance are more likely to have "basic" or "below basic" health literacy than "intermediate" or "proficient" health literacy.[14] A literature review prepared for the Kaiser Family Foundation revealed that health insurance is the single-most significant factor explaining racial disparities in having a usual source of care.[15,16]

Broadly speaking, the ACA intends to improve access to health insurance in four main ways: (1) the individual mandate, which requires all persons to have "qualifying or acceptable coverage"; (2) employer mandates requiring coverage for employees in businesses with more than 50 employees; (3) regional/state exchanges that allow individuals and small businesses to purchase coverage of varying benefit and cost, and choose from subsidized plans (for those up to the 400 percent of the federal poverty level, or FPL); and 4) the expansion of Medicaid eligibility to all individuals up to 133 percent of FPL. Additional provisions seek to broaden the scope and affordability of insurance coverage by, among other things: prohibiting insurance companies from rescinding coverage; extending dependent coverage for young adults until age 26; eliminating lifetime limits on coverage; regulating annual dollar limits on insurance coverage; and prohibiting the denial of coverage to children based on pre-existing conditions.

As many of those charged with implementing the ACA realize, none of these reforms will fully

---

[14] 2003 National Assessment of Adult Literacy (NAAL), National Center for Education Statistics, U.S. Department of Education

[15] Testimony of Marsha Lillie-Blanton, Dr.P.H., Senior Advisor on Race, Ethnicity, and Health Care, Henry J. Kaiser Family Foundation, before the House Ways and Means Subcommittee on Health. June 10, 2008.

[16] American College of Physicians. Racial and Ethnic Disparities in Health Care, Updated 2010. Philadelphia: American College of Physicians; 2010: Policy Paper.

succeed without efforts to make all of these opportunities understandable to the intended beneficiaries. These expansions must be accompanied by targeted efforts to enroll under-resourced populations. Given their inexperience with health coverage and the delivery system, these individuals will have greater difficulty with a number of its facets: understanding eligibility guidelines for various insurance programs; participating in the buy-in process of the exchange or high-risk pools; providing supplemental identification and citizenship documentation necessary for enrollment; understanding which services are covered; recognizing cost-sharing and premium responsibilities; and choosing a health care provider. All of these tasks require significant consumer education and assistance. Notably, one ACA provision calls for the development and utilization of uniform explanations of coverage documents and standardized definitions. This is an important mandate that could be strengthened with explicit linkages to health literacy.

The ACA also establishes an internet portal to help individuals and businesses interact with the insurance exchange. This tool will have to assist users in understanding eligibility guidelines for Medicaid/CHIP/Medicare/high-risk pools and subsidized private insurance. As such, the portal should contain easy-to-understand explanations in simple English, as well as be available in multiple languages. The ACA also requires that information presented by the national and regional exchanges be culturally and linguistically appropriate.

To be most effective, ACA requirements to make insurance and enrollment information consumer-friendly should extend beyond readable web and print materials to include media such as phone, television, radio, social media, and in-person outreach. Research shows that a higher percentage of adults with low literacy receive their information about health issues from radio and television than through written sources, the internet, or social contacts.[17] Use of community-based organizations, culturally specific media campaigns, *promotores,* and individual insurance brokers (many of whom will be displaced due to the exchanges) will drive effective enrollment of the highly diverse, newly eligible population. The economic recession has shown, for example, that affected families have turned first to community-based organizations for help with linking them to public assistance programs.[18] States can use specially allocated ACA funding for such local outreach and enrollment supports.

Medicaid Expansion. ACA law mandates that starting in 2014, Medicaid cover everyone under age 65 and 133 percent of FPL ($14,404 for one person in 2009). Accordingly, Medicaid could be serving upwards of 80 million Americans — or a quarter of the U.S. population — each year after 2014. Recent analyses suggest that this "expansion population" will likely: be racially and ethnically diverse; be predominantly childless adults; have high levels of substance abuse and prior jail involvement; and require integrated care management for complex physical and behavioral health needs.[19] It is fair to assume that health literacy would be a significant issue for this population, as current Medicaid beneficiaries face serious communication barriers related to limited literacy, language, culture, and disability.[20] Most new enrollees are unlikely to have had prior insurance,

[17] Kutner, M. et al The Health Literacy of America's Adults: Results from the 2003 National Assessment of Adult Literacy. Washington, DC: U.S.Department of Education, National Center for Education, 2006

[18] Kaiser Commission on Medicaid and the Uninsured. Optimizing Medicaid Enrollment: Perspectives on Strengthening Medicaid's Reach under Health Care Reform. Kaiser Family Foundation, Publication #8068. April 2010

[19] S. Somers, A. Hamblin, J. Verdier and V. Byrd. "Covering Low-Income Childless Adults in Medicaid: Experiences from Selected States." Center for Health Care Strategies. August 2010.

[20] Neuhauser L, Rothschild B, Graham C, Ivey SL, Konishi S (2009). Participatory design of mass health communication in three languages for seniors and people with disabilities on Medicaid. *American Journal of Public Health* 99(12): 2188-2195.

and thus will have limited knowledge about the Medicaid program, its services, and the complex administrative processes associated with enrollment and participation.

Simplifying Medicaid enrollment for diverse populations is not a new concept: the majority of states have some health literacy standards for their Medicaid programs. About 90 percent of all states have specific readability guidelines for Medicaid enrollment materials.[21] Of these, 67 percent call for at least a sixth-grade reading level or a range including, and 22 percent call for the level to be even lower. Ninety-six percent of states have simplified their enrollment forms, using easy-to-read language and repetition of key messages, such as when to use emergency care services. Eighty-two percent of states offer one-on-one enrollment assistance, and 72 percent provide onsite assistance at state agency offices, counseling sessions at local nonprofits and community centers, and/or a toll-free helpline.[22] Despite these efforts, many racial and ethnic minorities eligible for Medicaid or CHIP coverage — more than 80 percent of eligible uninsured African-American children and 70 percent of eligible uninsured Latino children — are still not enrolled.[23]

For current Medicaid beneficiaries who do not speak English or who have LEP, most states provide interpretive and translation services. The Centers for Medicare and Medicaid Services (CMS) has released readability guidelines for Medicaid print materials to states and has mandated certain contract requirements around communication standards for Medicaid managed care plans.[24] However, these guidelines lack strong enforcement or uniform oversight from any particular federal or state agency.

The following three ACA provisions, while not clearly linked to literacy, help further to simplify Medicaid eligibility determinations and streamline enrollment: (1) elimination of the asset test that many states still apply when determining Medicaid eligibility for adults, removing a common administrative burden and impediment to participation; (2) usage of a new, uniform method for determining income eligibility for most individuals (modified adjusted gross income, or MAGI); and (3) the expansion of the state option to presumptive eligibility determinations. The ACA also streamlines citizenship documentation requirements and electronic enrollment processes set forth by the Children's Health Insurance Program Reauthorization (CHIPRA) legislation in 2009.[25] To the extent that federal entities could provide monetary and technical assistance support for state health literacy efforts, Medicaid programs would be better able to effectively enroll and provide quality care to newly eligible, low-literacy populations in 2014 and beyond.

Individual Protections, Equity, and Special Populations

Individual Protections, Equity, and Special Populations	
Sample of Indirect Instances where Health Literacy could be addressed	
Section Number	**Provision Title**
Sec. 1557	Nondiscrimination

---

[21] Health Literacy Innovations, LLC. National Survey of Medicaid Guidelines for Health Literacy. 2003
[22] Matthews T, Sewell J. *State official's guide to health literacy*. Lexington, KY: Council of State Governments, 2002.
[23] American College of Physicians. Racial and Ethnic Disparities in Health Care, Updated 2010. Philadelphia: American College of Physicians; 2010: Policy Paper.
[24] Rosenbaum et al. *The Legality of Collecting and Disclosing Patient Race and Ethnicity Data*. George Washington University Department of Health Policy: 2006
[25] US Congress. H.R. 2: *Children's Health Insurance Program Reauthorization Act of 2009*. Pallone, F. Accessible at: http://www.govtrack.us/congress/bill.xpd?bill=h111-2

Sec. 4302	Understanding health disparities; data collection and analysis
Sec. 6301	Patient-Centered Outcomes Research
Sec. 10334	Minority health

The Insurance expansions in the ACA constitute significant steps toward universal coverage. All Americans up to a certain level of poverty (133 percent) will for the first time be entitled to health insurance. Protecting these lower-income individuals' right to health care is important to the successful implementation of the ACA. The law references the Civil Rights Act, the Education Amendments Act, the Age Discrimination Act, and the Rehabilitation Act. Section 1557's Non-Discrimination provision prevents exclusion of an individual from participation in or denial of benefits under any health program or activity.

The ACA also provides consumers with significant new protections, including the ability to choose a health plan that best suits their needs, to appeal a plan's to denial of coverage for needed services, and to select an available primary care provider of their choosing. Health plans are now required to communicate these patient protections in media that are "culturally and linguistically appropriate," and by extension, readable for those with low literacy levels. This term is used seven times in the legislation, including in references to: federal oral health and nutrition education programs; clinical depression centers of excellence; workforce training curricula; and the need for patient-centered delivery models to be culturally competent, i.e. sensitive to the beliefs, values, and cultural mores that influence how health care information is shared and received by individuals. Prior efforts of the HHS' Office of Civil Rights to set compliance standards for language aimed to improve access for those who have LEP and are already providing related regulations. But, there is no language in the ACA instructing this body or others to oversee the new "culturally and linguistically appropriate" obligations.

ACA law also requires the collection and reporting of data on race, ethnicity, sex, primary language, and disability status by all federally conducted and supported health care and public health programs (e.g., Medicare, Medicaid), activities, and surveys (including surveys conducted by the Bureau of Labor Statistics and the Bureau of the Census). It also urges the HHS to strengthen existing requirements that state Medicaid agencies collect race, ethnicity, and language data. The law specifies that existing Office of Management and Budget standards must be used, at a minimum, for recording race and ethnicity, and instructs the HHS to issue new standards for measuring sex, primary language, and disability status.

In 2000, the Office of Minority Health (OMH) developed National Standards on Culturally and Linguistically Appropriate Services (CLAS) to provide a common understanding and consistent definitions of culturally and linguistically appropriate services in health care. These standards were intended to be a practical framework for providers, payers, accreditation organizations, policymakers, health administrators, and educators. Post-reform health literacy efforts should make use of this resource, particularly since the OMH is gaining additional recognition in the law. The ACA establishes an OMH in every major agency within the HHS: AHRQ, CDC, CMS, FDA, Health Resources and Services Administration (HRSA), and Substance Abuse and Mental Health Services Administration (SAMHSA). These offices will be charged with evaluating the effectiveness of federal programs and targeted research to meet the needs of minority populations. Similarly, a newly created Patient Centered Outcomes Research Institute is tasked with conducting comparative effectiveness research, and ensuring that subpopulations, particularly communities of color, are represented in research designs.

The ACA's disparities agenda includes additional measures to support the rights and unique needs of certain populations. These include standardizing complaint forms for patients in nursing facilities; improving quality of care and protections for those in long-term care institutions; expanding aging and disability resource centers; providing dementia prevention and abuse training for personnel working in geriatric mental health; and appropriating funds for the Indian Health Care Improvement Act,[26] which supports the growth of the Native American health care force and innovative delivery models for rural populations and tribal organizations. Again, however, these provisions make no explicit link to health literacy.

---

[26] US Congress. S.1790: Indian Health Care Improvement Reauthorization and Extension Act of 2009. Dorgan, B. Accessible at: http://www.govtrack.us/congress/bill.xpd?bill=s111-1790

Workforce Development

Workforce Development	
Section Number	**Provision Title**
Direct Mentions of Health Literacy	
Sec. 5301	Training in Family Medicine, General Internal Medicine, General Pediatrics, and Physician Assistant- ship Presentation of Prescription Drug Benefit and Risk Information
Sample of Indirect Instances where Health Literacy could be addressed	
Sec. 5205	Allied health workforce recruitment and retention program
Sec. 5307	Cultural Competency, Prevention, and Public Health and Individuals With Disabilities Training
Sec. 5402	Health professions training for diversity
Sec. 5403	Interdisciplinary, community-based linkages
Sec. 5507	Demonstration project to address health professions workforce needs; extension of family-to-family health information centers
Sec. 5606	State grants to health care providers who provide services to a high percentage of medically under- served populations or other special populations

Within the next 40 years, people of color will make up the majority of the U.S. population.[27] Insurance reforms and expansion of coverage will bring to providers' offices new socially, culturally, and linguistically diverse patient populations, many of which are likely to have limited experience with the health system, difficulty communicating with practitioners, and complex
conditions that require effective self-management. There will be increased onus on health care
providers and their delivery system partners to be sensitive to the nuanced needs and potential
limitations of their patient populations. Not doing so could have major consequences for the patient's health, the physician's performance, and the payer's pocketbook.

Effectively communicating with low-literate patients is not an arcane skill: a survey of Federally
Qualified Health Centers, free clinics, and migrant health facilities found that when clinicians use
plain language, illustrations, and "talk back" methods, patient understanding, compliance, and
trust are greatly improved.[28] As it stands today, however, physicians are given little training in
this area during the course of their medical education,[29] and professionals who do receive a mod-
icum of training in this vein — community health workers and nurses, case managers, and public
health specialists, for example — lack recognition, funding, and inclusion in most physician-led
delivery teams. Other system issues such as pressure on provider time, use of singular modes of
communication, and cultural mismatch between provider and patient also contribute to subpar
delivery of health care services to low-literate patients.[30] Appropriately, the ACA legislation
pushes for improvement in the education and communications skills of a wide range of health

---

[27] U.S. Census Bureau. "Projected Population of the United States, by Race and Hispanic
Origin: 2000 to 2050. *http://www.census.gov/ipc/www/usinterimproj/natprojtab01a.pdf*
[28] Barret S.R et al. *Health Literacy Practices in Primary Care Settings: Examples
from the Field*. The Commonwealth Fund. 2008
[29] American College of Physicians. *Racial and Ethnic Disparities in Health Care, Updated 2010*. Philadelphia: American College of Physicians: 2010: Policy Paper
[30] Paasche-Orlow MK, Schillinger D, Green SM, Wagner EH. How healthcare systems can
begin to address the challenge of limited literacy. *Journal of General Internal Medicine*.
2006; 21(8): 884-887.

provider types, positioning workforce development as an important lever for establishing health care equity across diverse patient populations.

The ACA provides scholarships, grants, and loan repayment programs for health care professionals in medical fields such as primary care and mental health; offers continuing education support for those who serve minority, rural, and special populations; and improves medical school and health professions curricula in the areas of cultural competency and disabilities training. The ACA also seeks to increase the racial/ethnic diversity of health practitioners through educational grants and loan programs, and widens the array of professional and para-professionals available to patients through funding for training of community health workers, nurses, geriatric specialists, adolescent mental health providers, home care aides, and others.

Only one of these provisions — the primary care provider workforce training awards — explicitly mentions the term health literacy. But, other language related to cultural and linguistic appropriateness appears frequently, particularly as a condition of eligibility for the workforce grant opportunities.

Health Information

Health Information	
Section Number	**Provision Title**
Direct Mentions of Health Literacy	
Sec. 3507	Presentation of Prescription Drug Benefit and Risk Information
Sample of Indirect Instances where Health Literacy could be addressed	
Sec. 3305	Improved Information for Subsidy Eligible Individuals Reassigned to Prescription Drug and MA-PD Plans
Sec. 3503	Grants to implement medication management services in treatment of chronic disease
Sec. 4205	Nutrition labeling of standard menu items at chain restaurants
Sec. 10328	Improvement in Part D medication therapy management (MTM) programs

While the average piece of health care information is written at a 10th-grade reading level, the average American reads at only a fifth-grade level.[31] Numerous studies show that those with limited health literacy skills are at increased risk of misunderstanding medical information on product labels, manuals, package inserts, and nutrition labels.[32,33]

The ACA provisions on nutrition labeling, the presentation of prescription drug information, and medical management assistance are welcome. These provisions do not mandate health system-wide standards but recommend small-scale changes and building an evidence base for future implementation. They constitute an important step in acknowledging that health information, which is often dense, technical, and jargon-filled, must be digestible to the diverse consumers who are

---

[31] Rosales. 'Are Adequate Steps Being Taken to Address Health Literacy in this Country?" *Managed Care Outlook*. Volume 23, Number 11. Aspen Publishers: June 1, 2010
[32] Institute of Medicine, *Preventing Medication Errors: The Quality Chasm Series*, National Academies Press, 2006
[33] Weiss, Barry D., Mays, Mary Z., et al, "Quick assessment of literacy in primary care: The newest vital sign," *Annals of Family Medicine*, 3:514-522, 2005

trying to use it.

For instance, because of the high national prevalence of cardio-metabolic conditions, consumers are increasingly asked to control their diets. This requires them to be able to read and interpret labels that provide information on sugar, fat, salt, and cholesterol content. The difficulties in understanding nutrition and prescription drug information are heightened for those with "basic" and "below basic" levels of literacy.[34] These individuals have trouble finding pieces of information or numbers in a lengthy text, integrating multiple pieces of information in a document, or finding two or more numbers in a chart and performing a calculation.[35]

Elders and others with multiple chronic conditions are often given prescriptions for numerous medications by a mix of physical health and mental health providers, who may not communicate with each other about their prescription practices. This places the onus of medication reconciliation on the patient, whose literacy and numeracy skills might be compromised.

Complications around choice of plan eligibility and prescription drug reimbursement add other challenges for Part D Medicare beneficiaries. ACA provisions call for improved information for subsidy-eligible individuals reassigned to prescription drug and MA-PD plans, and put into place medication management programs for Part D seniors and chronic disease patients. These should help vulnerable beneficiaries with their health information demands. To be effective, these efforts should also focus on the verbal communications used by providers, pharmacists, and other dispensers of medication, to ensure that patients understand medication dosage, schedules, side effects and safety precautions.

Given the increasing presence of information technology in health communications, delivery and management, it will be important that this medium be accessible to low-literate, and low computer-literate users in particular. In several instances, the ACA promotes the use of the internet and web-based tools to disseminate health information and to communicate federal activities to a diverse consumer population. Some of these include:

- The "ombudsman" portal to facilitate enrollment into public and publicly subsidized insurance programs and the exchange;
- A website recommending prevention practices for specified chronic diseases and conditions;
- A web-based tool to create personalized prevention plans; and
- An internet portal for consumers to access health risk assessment tools.

Those designing these media should look to resources like the *Health Literacy Online Guide,*[36] a research-based how-to module developed by the HHS' Office of Disease Prevention and Health Promotion (ODPHP) to guide administrators, providers, and educators seeking to present information to low-literacy Americans using the web.

In terms of promoting the meaningful use of electronic health records (EHRs), there is little in the ACA that speaks to health literacy. However, health literacy advocates might note relevant re-

---

[34] The Joint Commission. *"What did the Doctor Say?: Improving Health Literacy to Protect Patient Safety.* Joint Commission: 2007.

[35] Berkman et. al. *Literacy and Health Outcomes.* Agency for Healthcare Research and Quality (AHRQ). Rockville, MD: 2004

[36] .S. Department of Health and Human Services, Office of Disease Prevention and Health Promotion. (2010). *Health literacy online: A guide to writing and designing easy-to-use health Web sites.* Washington, DC: Author.

quirements in the American Recovery and Reinvestment Act (ARRA) [37] legislation: (1) patients must be provided timely access (within 96 hours) to their electronic health information; (2) the EHR should be used to identify and provide patient-specific education resources; and (3) health care providers using an EHR must collect race and ethnicity data on their patients, using the OMB's classification standards.

---

[37] U.S. Congress. H.R.1: American Recovery and Reinvestment Act of 2009. Obey, D. Accessible at http://www.govtrack.us/congress/bill.xpd?bill=h111-1

Public Health, Health Promotion, and Prevention & Wellness

Public Health, Health Promotion, and Prevention & Wellness	
Section Number	Provision Title
Sec. 2951	Maternal, infant, and early childhood home visiting programs
Sec. 2953	Personal responsibility education
Sec. 4001	National Prevention, Health Promotion and Public Health Council
Sec. 4002	Prevention and Public Health Fund
Sec. 4003	Clinical and Community Preventive Services
Sec. 4004	Education and Outreach Campaign Regarding Preventive Benefits
Sec. 4102	Oral Healthcare Prevention Activities
Sec. 4103	Medicare coverage of annual wellness visit providing a personalized prevention plan
Sec. 4107	Coverage of comprehensive tobacco cessation services for pregnant women in Medicaid
Sec. 4108	Incentives for prevention of chronic diseases in Medicaid
Sec. 4201	Community transformation grants
Sec. 4202	Healthy Aging/Living Well for Medicare
Sec. 4206	Demonstration project concerning individualized wellness plan
Sec. 4301	Research on optimizing the delivery of public health services
Sec. 4303	CDC and employer-based wellness programs
Sec. 4306	Funding for childhood obesity demonstration project
Sec. 5313	Grants to Promote Positive Health Behaviors and Outcomes
Sec. 10408	Grants for small businesses to provide comprehensive workplace wellness programs
Sec. 10413	Young women's breast health awareness and support of young women diagnosed with breast cancer
Sec. 10501	National diabetes prevention program

ACA establishes a comprehensive framework for federal, community-based public health activities, including a coordinating council, a national strategy, and a national education and outreach
campaign. The legislation also addresses prevention and wellness at state, community, clinic, and
organizational levels. Specifically, it:

- Expands coverage of clinical preventive services under Medicare, Medicaid, and private
  health insurance;
- Encourages the development and expansion of personalized wellness programs by employers and insurers;

- Expands federal grantmaking and other public health activities directed at the prevention of disease risk factors such as obesity and tobacco use, with a focus on community transformation; and
- Supports evidence review processes to determine whether specific clinical (e.g. cancer screenings) and community-based prevention interventions (e.g. media campaigns) are effective.

Notably, the large national outreach and education undertaking to be led by the HHS and CDC will include a science-based media campaign; a chronic disease website to educate consumers; a web-based tool for individuals to create personalized prevention plans; and an internet portal with health risk assessment tools developed by academic entities. In addition, each state must design a public awareness campaign to educate Medicaid enrollees about the availability and coverage of preventive services, such as obesity-reduction programs for children and adults.

ACA also requires Medicaid health plans to cover tobacco cessation counseling and drug therapy for pregnant women. States that include a package of recommended preventive services (as set by the U.S. Preventive Services Task Force) for Medicaid-eligible adults will receive an enhanced federal match. Medicare Part B will be required to cover personalized prevention services for elders, including chronic disease testing and treatment, medication reconciliation, cognitive impairment assessments, and tailored wellness guidance. Other related programs authorized in the ACA that target specific populations and health gaps include: a national oral health education campaign; early motherhoold-child visiting programs; teenage personal responsibility grants; a national diabetes prevention program; childhood obesity-reduction initiatives; and centers for excellence in depression.

Although competencies around emergency preparedness and infectious disease are not a notable part of ACA's public health provisions, they should not be ignored during the implementation of national and community-based public health efforts. For example, individuals with compromised health literacy are likely less equipped to receive pertinent information or act expeditiously in the face of environmental disasters and pandemic disease outbreaks.[38,39]

Being healthy or learning how to become and stay healthy requires substantial self-activation, resources, willpower, and lifestyle modification. These are challenging for any patient, let alone one with low health literacy, who may encounter other structural barriers to good health. Such obstacles may include substandard housing; transportation difficulty; low job availability; poor educational opportunities; higher exposure to environmental toxins; involvement with violence and criminal justice; discrimination and socio-cultural marginalization; and limited access to fresh, healthy foods. These social problems and the circumstances of "place" have been shown to have a significant impact on the health of the underserved, many of whom also face low literacy.[40,41]

---

[38] Zarcadoolas,C., J. Boyer, A.Krishnaswami, & A. Rothenberg. (2007). "How usable are current GIS maps: communicating emergency preparedness to vulnerable populations?" Journal of Homeland Security and Emergency Management.

[39] Zarcadoolas, C., Pleasant, A. & Greer, D.S. (2006) *Advancing Health Literacy: A Framework for Understanding and Action.* San Francisco, CA: Jossey-Bass.

[40] Smedley, B. *Building stronger communities for better health: moving from science to policy to practice.* IOM Workshop: "Ten years later: how far have we come on reducing disparities?" 2010

[41] Andrulis et al. *Patient Protection and Affordable Care Act: Advancing Health Equity for Racially and Ethnically Diverse Populations.* Joint Center for Political and Economic Studies. Washington DC: July 2010

Innovations in Quality and the Delivery and Costs of Care

Innovations in Quality and the Delivery and Costs of Care	
Section Number	**Provision Title**
Direct Mentions of Health Literacy	
Sec. 3501	Health Care Delivery System Research; Quality Improvement Technical Assistance
Sec. 3506	Program to Facilitate Shared Decision-making
Sample of Indirect Instances where Health Literacy could be addressed	
Sec. 2703	State option to provide health homes for enrollees with chronic conditions
Sec. 3011	National strategy
Sec. 3012	Interagency Working Group on Health Care Quality
Sec. 3013	Quality measure development
Sec. 3014	Quality measurement
Sec. 3015	Data Collection; Public Reporting
Sec. 3021	Establishment of Center for Medicare and Medicaid Innovation within CMS
Sec. 3502	Grants or contracts to establish community health teams to support the patient-centered medical home
Sec. 3510	Patient navigator program
Sec. 10331	Public reporting of performance information
Sec. 10333	Community-based collaborative care networks

There is no dearth of provisions in the ACA focused on improving health care quality and reducing avoidable costs. The legislation identifies patient-centeredness, safety, efficiency, and equity as both vehicles for and by-products of the quality effort. Except for two mentions of health literacy in provisions regarding shared decision-making programs and dissemination of delivery system research, health literacy is not explicitly featured in the bill's language on quality. However, adults with low health literacy average six percent more hospital visits, remain in the hospital two days longer and have annual health care costs four times higher than those with proficient health literacy skills.[42] As such, literacy should be a core consideration in discussions of quality improvement, health delivery redesign, and cost-reduction.

The legislation uses three broad mechanisms to address quality: (1) a national approach that identifies an umbrella strategy, establishes a federal-level, inter-agency quality workgroup, sets an agenda for measurement, and develops metrics; (2) delivery system redesign through efforts targeting improved care coordination and new patient-centered care models such as the medical home; and (3) the reduction of cost through increased payer and provider accountability across private and public programs (e.g., pay-for-performance incentives and value-based purchasing structures).

---

[42] Partnership for Clear Health Communication at the National Patient Safety Foundation. *What is Health Literacy?* Ask Me 3. *Accessible at:* http://www.npsf.org/askme3/PCHC/what_is_health.php

Health literacy issues should be represented in the ACA-mandated inter-agency quality workgroup to be convened by the President, and in the development of the national quality strategy (i.e., readability standards for all federal health program communications). Quality measure development and endorsement efforts that will be spearheaded by AHRQ and CMS should gauge national health literacy trends and their implications, as well as explore how new measures that identify and stratify low-literacy risk groups can be used to improve care at the community, provider, plan, and hospital levels. The support for public reporting mechanisms in ACA may also provide consumers with better, more readable information about the performance of their health system, enabling more informed health care choices.

Many of the objectives of quality improvement — avoiding waste in the system; reducing the over- and underuse of medications, diagnostic tests, and therapies; and improving patient safety — depend on the patient's ability to be an informed and active player in his or her care. For low-literate populations, interacting with physicians, complying with medical guidance, and managing the disparate demands of multiple providers in fragmented delivery systems is that much more challenging.

Other quality components of the ACA that ensure patient-centeredness, such as the shared decision-making program and patient navigator services, should also resonate with health literacy advocates. Regional collaborative networks, the primary care extension hubs, health homes in Medicaid, and the use of community health teams to support the medical home, would all be strengthened by concerted attention to patients with low literacy, particularly those managing complex, co-morbid physical and mental health conditions. Estimates suggest that 75 percent of those with chronic conditions have low levels of health literacy.[43]

One of the most promising windows of opportunity among the quality-oriented provisions is the newly created Center for Medicare and Medicaid Innovation (CMI) within CMS. CMI will fund demonstration programs that research, test, and expand innovations in payment and delivery system improvement pilots. Given the prevalence of low literacy among individuals in publicly financed care, particularly people with disabilities in Medicaid and those dually eligible for Medicaid and Medicare,[44] this could be a prime opportunity to test health literacy innovations among high-risk populations such as pregnant women or elders with multiple medications. Such demonstrations could convey to federal and state policymakers the mediating power of health literacy to improve quality and reduce costs. This could also help demonstrate the business case for further investments in health literacy by health plans and accountable care organizations serving these populations.

Given the evidence base around populations disproportionately affected by low health literacy, Medicaid, Medicare, and Veterans Administration programs may present the best targets of opportunity for making the case. The Veterans Administration is a closed system with considerable data capacity, but might pose problems for generalizability; while Medicare is still largely a fee-for-service system, which provides few leverage points for concerted action. The 7.5 million individuals dually enrolled in Medicaid and Medicare could benefit from health literacy interventions given their age and complex health needs, but these "duals" are generally not in integrated care management programs that have enormous incentives to prevent the exacerbation of illness

---

[43] Hsu. *The Health Literacy of U.S. Adults Across GED Credential Recipients, High School Graduates, and Non-High School Graduates.* American Council on Education. GED Testing Service: 2008.
[44] Baker et. Al. Health Literacy and Mortality Among Elderly Persons. *Arch Intern Med* 167(14):1503-1509. 2007.

and disability associated with low health literacy. However, 71 percent of Medicaid's 60 million beneficiaries are enrolled in managed care;[45] as the nation's largest purchaser of health care, it could use its leverage to promote innovations in this arena. Medicaid managed care organizations already have the incentives to address health literacy, especially for those with complex conditions. But, to date, none have demonstrated that by using readily available and easy-to-administer literacy assessment tools (e.g., the short TOHFLA). They could identify and stratify a high-risk population with low literacy skills and design an intervention to help them manage their conditions- — consequently avoiding costly exacerbations, hospitalizations and institutionalizations.

Best Practices

"What Are My Medi-Cal Choices?"

Health Research for Action (HRA), a center at UC Berkeley's School of Public Health, was funded by the California Department of Health Care Services to create easy-to-read and understandable information for seniors and people with disabilities on Medi-Cal, about their Medi-Cal choices. This specific population could choose between Regular Medi-Cal (also known as Fee for Service) and Medi-Cal Managed Care Plans. The goals of this project were to:

1. Use participatory research to develop a guidebook that informed seniors and people with disabilities on Medi-Cal about their unique Medi-Cal choices.
2. Promote informed choice between Medi-Cal fee for service and Medi-Cal Managed Care delivery systems.

HRA conducted extensive formative research to understand how seniors and people with disabilities learn and make decisions about their Medi-Cal delivery options. Findings informed HRA's development of a draft consumer guidebook called *"What Are My Medi-Cal Choices?"* in English, Spanish, and Chinese. The formative research used a participatory model where beneficiaries and other stakeholders were consulted in the content and layout of the guidebook. HRA conducted 51 key informant interviews with stakeholders as well as extensive qualitative research with Medi-Cal beneficiaries including 24 one-on-one interviews, 18 focus groups, and 36 one-on-one usability tests. This formative research was conducted in English, Spanish, Mandarin, Cantonese, and American Sign Language. Formative research findings showed that that English-, Spanish- and Chinese-speaking Medi-Cal recipients who are seniors or people with disabilities had very little knowledge about their Medi-Cal choices and negative attitudes about managed care health plans. Several areas of unmet information needs and primary areas of concern for SPD beneficiaries when faced with Medi-Cal choices were also identified. In addition to the above formative research, an advisory group that included disability advocates, managed care plan representatives, health care providers, policymakers, and Medi-Cal beneficiaries provided guidance and feedback on the research, guidebook, the dissemination process, and complementary interventions.

The Department of Health Care Services disseminated the guidebook through a direct mailing to beneficiaries in the target population and via partner organizations. The final guidebook was developed in 12 threshold languages, plus alternative formats including Braille (English and Spanish only) and audio, including MP3, cassette, and CD (all 12 languages).

HRA conducted a multi-lingual mixed-methods evaluation of the final guidebook including 10 focus groups, 28 stakeholder interviews, and a randomized control trial telephone survey. At six weeks post-dissemination, the intervention group showed significantly higher increases in knowledge, confidence, positive attitudes about, and intentions to consider changing to a Medi-Cal health plan than did the control group. Overall, the findings provided strong evidence that the guidebook was an effective and low-cost way to improve reci-

---

[45] Medicaid Managed Care Penetration Rates by State as of June 30, 2008, Centers for Medicare and Medicaid Services, U.S. Department of Health and Human Services, special data request, August 2009.

pients' abilities to make more informed Medi-Cal choices.

In 2008, the Institute for Healthcare Advancement jointly awarded HRA and the DHCS the national first place award for Health Literacy for their work on the consumer guidebook.

III. Conclusion

The ACA is not a landmark piece of legislation for health literacy, but with its attention to increased coverage, quality improvement and cost reduction, it creates opportunities for bringing cultural competency, disparities, and health literacy to the fore. It establishes momentum for investments in innovation among state agencies, payers, providers, regulators, advocacy groups, and others to improve care in many ways, including patient-centered high quality care. Organizations promoting health literacy will not be armed with forceful legislative or with regulatory mandates or with designated resources, so they will have to continue to find ways to make the case for greater investment and action by both public and private stakeholders in our health care system.

The ACA does create opportunities for driving home the importance of health literacy in all of the key domains of health and health care identified earlier:

1. *The Coverage Expansion*: Establishing what is essentially universal coverage for 16 million Americans up to 133 percent of FPL and subsidized insurance options for another 16 million low income Americans will only be successful if the newly eligible individuals can understand their options and navigate the enrollment process.
2. *Equity*: Moving toward universal coverage and creating the same "floor" for all of our lowest-income populations should help address some of the fundamental disparities in access to care in this country, but as the legislation underscores, that will depend on the attention our health care delivery system pays to cultural differences, language, and by extension, literacy.
3. *Workforce*: The provider training provisions in ACA related to disparities, cultural competency, and patient-centeredness all present opportunities for bringing greater attention to health literacy.
4. *Health care Information*: From medication management to provider performance rating, patient information must be presented at reading and numeracy levels accessible to millions of Americans with low literacy skills.
5. *Public Health and* Wellness: The preparation and presentation (whether in print, electronically, or otherwise) of consumer information on issues ranging from wellness to emergency preparedness must be done with low literacy in mind.
6. *Quality* Improvement: The ACA's emphasis on developing, testing and spreading best practices for improving quality and reducing costs presents many new opportunities for making the case for investments in health literacy.

IV. Appendices[46]

Appendix A: Summary of ACA Provisions with Potential Implications for Health Literacy

Insurance Reform, Outreach, and Enrollment

Sec. 1002. Health insurance consumer information. The Secretary shall award grants to States to enable them (or the Exchange) to establish, expand, or provide support for offices of health insurance consumer assistance or health insurance ombudsman programs. These independent offices will assist consumers with filing complaints and appeals, educate consumers on their rights and responsibilities, and collect, track, and quantify consumer problems and inquiries.

Sec. 1103. Immediate information that allows consumers to identify affordable coverage options. Establishes an Internet portal for beneficiaries to easily access affordable and four comprehensive coverage options. This information will include eligibility, availability, premium rates, cost sharing, and the percentage of total premium revenues spent on health care, rather than administrative expenses, by the issuer. Section 10102 clarifies that the internet portal shall be available to small businesses and shall contain information on coverage options available to small businesses.

Sec. 1311. Affordable choices of health benefit plans. Requires the Secretary to award grants, available until 2015, to States for planning and establishment of American Health Benefit Exchanges. By 2014, requires States to establish an American Health Benefit Exchange that facilitates the purchase of qualified health plans and includes a SHOP Exchange for small businesses.

Sec. 1401. Refundable tax credit providing premium assistance for coverage under a qualified health plan. Amends the Internal Revenue Code to provide tax credits to assist with the cost of health insurance premiums.

Sec. 1413. Streamlining of procedures for enrollment through an Exchange and State Medicaid, CHIP, and health subsidy programs. Requires the Secretary to establish a system for the residents of each State to apply for enrollment in, receive a determination of eligibility for participation in, and continue participation in, applicable State health subsidy programs. The system will ensure that if any individual applying to an Exchange is found to be eligible for Medicaid or a State children's health insurance program (CHIP), the individual is enrolled for assistance under such plan or program.

Sec. 1513. Shared responsibility for employers. As amended by the *Reconciliation Act*, requires an employer with at least 50 full-time employees that does not offer coverage and has at least one full-time employee receiving a premium assistance tax credit to make a payment of $2,000 per full-time employee. Includes the number of full-time equivalent employees for purposes of de-

---

[46] Adapted from the following sources:

Communication with Sara Rosenbaum (Aug – Sept 2010). Hirsh Professor and Chair of the Health Policy Department at George Washington University.

Democratic Policy Committee, United States Senate. *Affordable Care Act: Section-by-Section Analysis with Changes Made by Title X and Reconciliation*. Updated September 17, 2010. Accessible at: http://dpc.senate.gov/dpcissue-sen_health_care_bill.cfm.

Williams E. and Redhead C. *Public Health, Workforce, Quality, and Related Provisions in the Patient Protection and Affordable Care Act (PPACA)*. Congressional Research Service (CRS) Report for Congress. 7-5700. June 2010. Accessible at http://www.crs.gov.

tion. Authorizes funding to geriatric education centers to support training in geriatrics, chronic care management, and long-term care for faculty in health professions schools and family caregivers; develop curricula and best practices in geriatrics; expand the geriatric career awards to advanced practice nurses, clinical social workers, pharmacists, and psychologists; and establish traineeships for individuals who are preparing for advanced education nursing degrees in geriatric nursing.

Sec. 5307. Cultural competency, prevention, and public health and individuals with disabilities training. Reauthorizes and expands programs to support the development, evaluation, and dissemination of model curricula for cultural competency, prevention, and public health proficiency and aptitude for working with individuals with disabilities training for use in health professions schools and continuing education programs.

Sec. 5309. Nurse education, practice, and retention grants. Awards grants to nursing schools to strengthen nurse education and training programs and to improve nurse retention.

Sec. 5313. Grants to promote the community health workforce. Authorizes the Secretary to award grants to States, public health departments, clinics, hospitals, Federally Qualified Health Centers (FQHCs), and other nonprofits to promote positive health behaviors and outcomes in medically underserved areas through the use of community health workers. Community health workers offer interpretation and translation services, provide culturally appropriate health education and information, offer informal counseling and guidance on health behaviors, advocate for individual and community health needs, and provide some direct primary care services and screenings.

Sec. 5316. Rural physician training grants. As added by Section 10501, establishes a grant program for medical schools to recruit and train medical students to practice medicine in underserved rural communities.

Sec. 5317. Demonstration grants for family nurse practitioner training programs. As added by Section 10501, establishes a training demonstration program that supports recent Family Nurse Practitioner graduates in primary care for a 12-month period in FQHCs and nurse-managed health clinics. The demonstration is authorized from 2011 through 2014

Sec. 5401. Centers of excellence. The Centers of Excellence program, which develops a minority applicant pool to enhance recruitment, training, academic performance and other supports for minorities interested in careers in health, is reauthorized.

Sec. 5402. Health professions training for diversity. Provides scholarships for disadvantaged students who commit to work in medically underserved areas as primary care providers, and expands loan repayments for individuals who will serve as faculty in eligible institutions.

Sec. 5403. Interdisciplinary, community-based linkages. Authorizes funding to establish community-based training and education grants for Area Health Education Centers and Programs Supports two programs targeting individuals from urban and rural medically underserved communities, who are seeking careers in the health professions.

Sec. 5507. Demonstration project to address health professions workforce needs; extension of family-to-family health information centers. Establishes a demonstration grant program through competitive grants to provide aid and supportive services to low-income individuals with the opportunity to obtain education and training for occupations in the health care field that pay well and are expected to experience labor shortages or be in high demand. The demonstration grant is to serve low-income persons including recipients of assistance under State Temporary Assistance for Needy Families (TANF) programs.

Sec. 5602. Negotiated rulemaking for development of methodology and criteria for designating medically underserved populations and health professions shortage areas. Directs the Secretary, in consultation with stakeholders, to establish a comprehensive methodology and criteria for designating medically underserved populations and Health Professional Shortage Areas.

Sec. 5606. State grants to health care providers who provide services to a high percentage of medically underserved populations or other special populations. As added by Section 10501, creates a grant program to support health care providers who treat a high percentage of medically underserved populations.

Sec 9024. Health professionals State loan repayment tax relief. As added by Section 10908, excludes from gross income payments made under any State loan repayment or loan forgiveness program that is intended to provide for the increased availability of health care services in underserved or health professional shortage areas.

Health Information

Sec. 3305. Improved information for subsidy-eligible individuals reassigned to prescription drug plans and MA–PD plans. Requires HHS, beginning in 2011, to transmit formulary and coverage determination information to subsidy-eligible beneficiaries who have been automatically reassigned to a new Part D low-income subsidy plan.

Sec. 3503. Grants to implement medication management services in treatment of chronic disease. Creates a program to support medication management services by local health providers.

Sec. 3507. Presentation of prescription drug benefit and risk information. Requires the Food and Drug Administration to evaluate and determine if the use of drug fact boxes which would clearly communicate drug risks and benefits and support clinician and patient decision making in advertising and other forms of communication for prescription medications is warranted.

Sec. 4205. Nutrition labeling of standard menu items at chain restaurants. Stipulates that a restaurant that is part of a chain with 20 or more locations doing business under the same name are required to disclose calories on the menu board and in a written form, as well as provide customers with additional nutritional information upon request.

Sec. 10328. Improvement in Part D medication therapy management programs. Requires Part D prescription drug plans to include a comprehensive review of medications and a written summary of the review as part of their medication therapy management programs.

Public Health, Health Promotion, and Prevention & Wellness

Sec. 2951. Maternal, infant, and early childhood home visiting programs. Provides funding to States, tribes, and territories to develop and implement one or more evidence-based Maternal, Infant, and Early Childhood Visitation model(s). Models aimed at reducing infant and maternal mortality and its related causes.

Sec. 2953. Personal responsibility education. Provides $75 million per year through FY2014 for Personal Responsibility Education grants to States for programs to educate adolescents on both abstinence and contraception for prevention of teenage pregnancy and sexually transmitted infections, including HIV/AIDS. Funding is also available for 1) innovative teen pregnancy prevention strategies and services to high-risk, vulnerable, and culturally under-represented populations, 2) allotments to Indian tribes and tribal organizations, and 3) research and evaluation, training, and technical assistance.

Sec. 4001. National Prevention, Health Promotion and Public Health Council. Creates an interagency council dedicated to promoting healthy policies at the federal level. The Council will establish a national prevention and health promotion strategy and develop interagency working relationships to implement the strategy.

Sec. 4002. Prevention and Public Health Fund. Establishes a Fund to provide an expanded and sustained national investment in prevention and public health programs to improve health and help restrain the rate of growth in private and public sector health care costs.

Sec. 4003. Clinical and community preventive services. Expands the efforts of, and improves the coordination between the U.S. Preventive Services Task Force and the Community Preventive Services Task Force. The latter uses a public health perspective to review the evidence of effectiveness of population-based preventive services such as tobacco cessation, increasing physical activity and preventing skin cancer, and develops recommendations for their use.

Sec. 4103. Medicare coverage of annual wellness visit providing a personalized prevention plan. Provides coverage under Medicare, with no co-payment or deductible, for an annual wellness visit and personalized prevention plan services.

Sec. 4107. Coverage of comprehensive tobacco cessation services for pregnant women in Medicaid. States would be required to provide Medicaid coverage for counseling and pharmacotherapy to pregnant women for cessation of tobacco use

Sec. 4108. Incentives for prevention of chronic diseases in Medicaid. The Secretary would award grants to States to provide incentives for Medicaid beneficiaries to participate in programs promoting healthy lifestyles.

Sec. 4201. Community transformation grants. Authorizes the Secretary to award competitive grants to eligible entities for programs that promote individual and community health and prevent incidence of chronic disease.

Sec. 4202. Healthy aging, living well; evaluation of community-based prevention and wellness programs for Medicare beneficiaries. The goal of this program is to improve the health status of the pre-Medicare-eligible population to help control chronic disease and reduce Medicare costs. The CDC will provide grants to States or large local health departments to conduct pilot programs in the 55-to-64 year old population. Pilot programs would evaluate chronic disease risk factors, conduct evidence-based public health interventions, and ensure that individuals identified with chronic disease or at-risk for chronic disease receive clinical treatment to reduce risk. Pilot programs will be evaluated for success in controlling Medicare costs in the community. Additionally, the Centers for Medicare & Medicaid Services (CMS) will conduct a comprehensive assessment of community-based disease self-management programs that help control chronic diseases. The Secretary will then develop a plan for improving access to such services for Medicare beneficiaries.

Sec. 4206. Demonstration project concerning individualized wellness plan. This pilot program provides at-risk populations who utilize community health centers with a comprehensive risk-factor assessment and individualized wellness plan to reduce risk factors for preventable conditions.

Sec. 4301. Research on optimizing the delivery of public health services. The Secretary, through the Director of CDC, shall provide funding for research in the area of public health services and systems. Research shall examine best practices relating to prevention, analyze the translation of interventions from academic institutions to clinics and communities, and identify effective strategies for delivering public health services in real-world settings.

Sec. 4303. CDC and employer-based wellness programs. Requires the CDC to study and evaluate best employer-based wellness practices and provide an educational campaign and technical assistance to promote the benefits of worksite health promotion to employers.

Sec. 4306. Funding for childhood obesity demonstration project. Appropriates $25 million for a demonstration project to develop a comprehensive and systematic model for reducing childhood obesity, which the Secretary must initiate under the Children's Health Insurance Program Reauthorization Act of 2009.

Sec. 10408. Grants for small businesses to provide comprehensive workplace wellness programs. Authorizes an appropriation of $200 million to give employees of small businesses access to comprehensive workplace wellness programs.

Sec. 10413. Young women's breast health awareness and support of young women diagnosed with breast cancer. Directs the Secretary of HHS to develop a national education campaign for young women and health care professionals about breast health and risk factors for breast cancer. Supports prevention research activities at the Centers for Disease Control and Prevention (CDC) on breast cancer in younger women.

Sec. 10501. National diabetes prevention program. Establishes a national diabetes prevention program at the CDC. State, local, and tribal public health departments and non-profit entities can use funds for community-based prevention activities, training and outreach, and evaluation.

Innovations in Quality and the Delivery and Costs of Care

Sec. 2703. State option to provide health homes for enrollees with chronic conditions. Provides States the option of enrolling Medicaid beneficiaries with chronic conditions into a health home. Health homes would be composed of a team of health professionals and would provide a comprehensive set of medical services, including care coordination.

Sec. 3011. National strategy. Requires the Secretary to establish and update annually a national strategy to improve the delivery of health care services, patient health outcomes, and population health. Establishes, not later than January 1, 2011, a federal health care quality internet website.

Sec. 3012. Interagency Working Group on Health Care Quality. Requires the President to convene a working group comprising federal agencies to collaborate on the development and dissemination of quality initiatives consistent with the national strategy.

Sec. 3013. Quality measure development. Authorizes $75 million over five years for the development of quality measures at Agency for Healthcare Research and Quality (AHRQ) and the Centers for Medicare and Medicaid Services (CMS). Measures must be consistent with the national strategy. As amended by Section 10303, requires the Secretary to develop and publicly report on patient outcomes measures.

Sec. 3014. Quality measurement. Provides $20 million to support the endorsement and use of endorsed quality and efficiency measures by the HHS Secretary for use in Medicare, reporting performance information to the public, and in health care programs.

Sec. 3015. Data Collection; Public Reporting. Requires the Secretary to collect and aggregate consistent data on quality and resource use measures from information systems used to support health care delivery to implement the public reporting of performance information.

Sec. 3021. Establishment of Center for Medicare and Medicaid Innovation within CMS. The purpose of the Center will be to research, develop, test, and expand innovative payment and delivery arrangements to improve the quality and reduce the cost of care provided to patients in each program.

Sec. 3501. Health care delivery system research; Quality improvement technical assistance. Builds on AHRQ's Center for Quality Improvement and Patient Safety to support research, technical assistance and process implementation grants. Grants funded will identify, develop, evaluate, disseminate, and provide training in innovative methodologies and strategies for quality improvement practices in the delivery of health care services.

Sec. 3502. Grants or contracts to establish community health teams to support the patient-centered medical home. Creates a program to establish and fund the development of community health teams to support the development of medical homes by increasing access to comprehensive, community based, coordinated care.

Sec. 3506. Program to facilitate shared decision-making. Establishes a program at HHS for the development, testing, and disseminating of educational tools to help patients, caregivers, and authorized representatives understand their treatment options.

Sec. 3510. Patient navigator program. Reauthorizes demonstration programs to provide patient navigator services within communities to assist patients overcome barriers to health services.

Sec. 10330. Modernizing computer and data systems of CMS to support improvements in care delivery. Requires the Secretary of HHS to develop a plan to modernize the computer and data systems of CMS to support improvements in care delivery.

Sec. 10331. Public reporting of performance information. Requires the Secretary of HHS to develop a "Physician Compare" website where Medicare beneficiaries can compare scientifically sound measures of physician quality and patient experience measures.

Sec. 10333. Community-based collaborative care networks. Provides grants to develop networks of providers to deliver coordinated care to low-income populations.

Appendix B: Instances of "Culturally and Linguistically Appropriate" in the ACA

Culturally and Linguistically Appropriate	
Section Number	**Provision Title**
Sec. 1311.	Affordable choices of health benefit plans.
Sec. 2715.	Development and utilization of uniform explanation of coverage documents and standardized definitions.
Sec. 2719.	Appeals process.
Sec. 4102.	Oral healthcare prevention activities.
Sec. 5313.	Grants to promote the community health workforce.
Sec. 5405.	Primary care extension program.
Sec. 10410.	Centers of excellence for depression

D

Health Literacy and the Health Reform: Where Do Children Fit In?

Lee M. Sanders, M.D., M.P.H.
Comments for Institute of Medicine
Workshop on Health Literacy and Health Reform
November 10, 2010

LIFE-COURSE PERSPECTIVE ON HEALTH LITERACY

At least 1 in 3 parents of young children have limited health literacy skills. Limited health literacy is independently associated with each of the major child-health objectives in *Healthy People 2010*. Two recent reviews suggest that the strongest and most consistent associations are those between a mother's health literacy and her own mental health (itself a modifiable determinant of child health), between a mother's health literacy and her child's access to needed care, and between an adolescent's health literacy and her/his likelihood to engage in risky health behaviors.

The Affordable Care Act provides several opportunities for state and federal agencies, alongside health plans and community-based organizations, to address these literacy-related disparities in child health, but doing so will require a life-course perspective that reaches from infancy through old age. (See Figure D-1.) At the individual level, imagine the following scenario: Ms. Garcia is a second-generation, legal immigrant from Central America; she has limited English proficiency, less than a 7th-grade education, works as a hotel janitor, and has just given birth to her first child, Zoe. During infancy and early childhood, the educational system provides Zoe access to a high-quality preschool (building Zoe's emergent-literacy skills) and her mother access to adult basic education (building Ms. Garcia's job prospects), and the health system provides Zoe with comprehensive and continuous health insurance (allowing access to needed preventive and acute care), an intensive nurse home visiting program (building Ms. Garcia's health literacy skills), and a family-centered

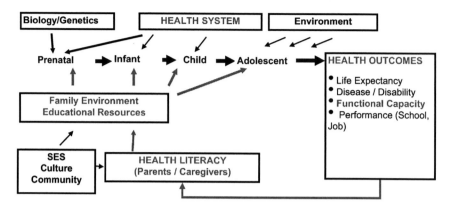

FIGURE D-1 Life course perspective on health literacy.
SOURCE: Sanders, L.M., adapted from Halfon, N., Hochstein, M. *Milbank Quarterly* 2002; 80(3):433.

medical home (embracing needed medical, dental, nutritional, and psychosocial support services). During the school-age years and adolescence, the educational system provides Zoe an effective curriculum that integrates developmentally appropriate health-behavior content within her reading, math and science curricula, and the health system continues to provide access to the family-centered medical home. As a health-literate adult, Zoe effectively accesses and uses written and electronic health information, and she serves as an effective advocate for her own health, for her children's health, and for her grandchildren's health.

At the population-health and public-policy level, this life-course perspective suggests that improving the nation's health will require coordinated investments from educational and health systems to support the health literacy skills of individuals as they mature from newborn citizens to senior citizens.

RECOMMENDATIONS

In response to the Affordable Care Act, the Institute of Medicine's Health Literacy Roundtable could best improve the ACA's attention to this life-course perspective on child health by focusing discussions on community-based funding, advocacy, and research on the following priorities:

1. *To Extend Coverage to All Children*: **Simplify the CHIP and Medicaid Enrollment Process.**

2. *To Improve the Quality of Child Health Care*: Target and Tailor Medical-Home Services for Low-Literacy Parents of Children with Complex Chronic Illnesses.
3. *To Improve Child Medication Safety*: Promote National Standards for Safe-Use Labeling of Pediatric Liquid Medication.
4. *To Improve the Skills of the Pediatric Workforce*: Advocate for Effective Health Literacy Training as a Required Competency for Post-Graduate Training in Pediatrics.

1. EXTENDING HEALTH-INSURANCE COVERAGE TO ALL CHILDREN

Background. At least 9 million U.S. children are uninsured, and of those, at least 5 million are eligible for public insurance, including Medicaid and the Children's Health Insurance Program (CHIP). Rates of uninsured children are highest in under-resourced communities with the highest prevalence of low-literacy and limited English-proficiency adults. Adjusting for income, age, and English-language proficiency, a recent analysis of the NAAL indicates that children of caregivers with low health literacy are significantly more likely to be uninsured.[14] These children are also more likely to have unmet health care needs,[26] to make more unnecessary visits to the emergency room,[27] and to be enrolled in other eligible social programs (e.g., WIC, TANF). (Pati S, et al. Influence of Maternal Health Literacy on Child Participation in Social Welfare Programs: The Philadelphia Experience. Am J Public Health. 2010;100:1662-1665.)

Many parents are unable to understand and complete child-health-insurance enrollment documents, and for state programs like Medicaid and CHIP, many more are impeded by the cumbersome enrollment process. On a single item from the National Assessment of Adult Literacy, nearly 2 in 3 were not able to fill in the name and birth date in the appropriate places on a health-insurance form. In 2007, 26 states used enrollment forms for CHIP too complex for most U.S. adults to understand. Their written instructions were written above the 10th-grade level, and the forms themselves were assessed as too difficult to complete by independent standards ("Suitability Assessment of Materials") and CHIP-legislated standards.[19] While the complexity of enrollment forms is clearly a significant enrollment barrier for low-literacy families with CHIP or Medicaid-eligible children,[97] a recent Urban Institute study suggested that the barriers to CHIP enrollment were myriad, including cumbersome enrollment eligibility screening processes, narrow enrollment periods, and under-resourced state outreach efforts. In response to Children's Health Insurance Reauthorization Act (CHIPRA) incentives—only 17 states have implemented "eligibility simplification efforts" (e.g., continuous eligibility, elimination of the face-to-face interview, presumptive eligibility for newborns born to Medicaid-insured mothers, and use of a bundled eligibility for multiple programs). To date, these efforts have resulted in enrolling at least 1 million children in CHIP or Medicaid.

ACA-Related Recommendations. ACA and CHIPRA provide ample opportunity to expand insurance coverage for all children in the United States. Bridging literacy-related barriers is made possible by three ACA provisions (Sec. 1413, 2715, and 3306), which complement the CHIPRA incentives for simplifying the enrollment process. ACA and CHIPRA afford all states the funding to do the following:

A. *Conduct low-literacy CHIP-enrollment outreach campaigns, targeting communities with the highest prevalence of low literacy skills among adult caregivers of young children.* Community-based organizations are essential to the success of these campaigns, and they should have easy access to national resources, such as ARHQ's Health Literacy Toolkit, to help reach and communicate with low-literacy communities. Easy-to-understand, single-page explanations of ACA should be developed. (See Box D-1 for draft language.)

B. *Assure that paper and web-based application forms for CHIP and Medicaid are written at or below established suitability and grade-level standards.* In accordance with the Plain Language Act, specific deadlines, designated officials at state and federal levels, and reporting provisions may be issued by HHS to assure that these standards are met.

C. *Bundle the eligibility assessment for all maternal and child health programs* (e.g., WIC, SNAP, school-lunch program, CHIP, Medicaid for children, and Medicaid for adult caregivers of eligible children). Disseminated established state-based best practices (developed in the early months of CHIPRA simplification efforts), Centers for Medicaid and Medicare (CMS) could provide models for such bundled eligibility and enrollment processes to all states. CMS and their state-based counterparts could encourage interagency agreements to facilitate "presumptive eligibility" across health, nutritional, and social-service programs.

D. *Assess eligibility for all maternal and child-health programs at school entry and at school health clinics.* Public-school enrollment and orientation, as well as enrollment activities for Head Start and other federally-subsidized child-care centers, should be designated as "priority portals" for the Health Insurance Exchanges established by the ACA. This may provide additional opportunity to guarantee insurance coverage, not just for school-aged children but also for their parents, grandparents and other adult caregivers.

BOX D-1
What the Health Reform Act Means for Your Child

1. It makes sure that your child has health insurance.

2. It makes sure that your child will get immunizations and regular health checks.

3. It makes sure that your child has a regular place to go to get medical care.

If your child is over age 18, it allows your child to stay on your health insurance plan until age 26.

In some states and counties:
1. If your child was just born, the Act may provide a specially trained nurse to visit your home. The nurse will help you get through those difficult first few weeks.

2. If your child has a chronic medical or behavioral problem, a specialized nurse will help you manage the problem at home and at school.

More information at www.kidshealth.org

2. IMPROVING THE QUALITY OF HEALTH CARE FOR ALL CHILDREN

Background. Improving health care quality for all children will likely require health system changes that provide each child with a Family-Centered Medical Home, an evidence-based system of care that was originally developed to attend to the needs of children with complex chronic conditions.[2,4,73] The key components of a family-centered medical home are continuous access to comprehensive, culturally effective, and coordinated care that meets the health and developmental needs of the child and her/his family. In practice, this often means minor restructuring to a hospital or primary care system that facilitates 24/7 telephone access and a care coordinator (nurse, parent, or community health worker) to serve as a patient navigator. Nurse home-visiting programs, normally implemented in the first year after a child's birth, help support the family-centered medical home by providing mothers with individualized, home-based education on infant care, increased access to maternal and child primary care services, and increased access to other social services (e.g., breastfeeding and nutritional support, maternal mental health services, and child developmental screening and intervention services). Children's hospitals, academic medical systems, and pediatric managed-care organizations, and have led large-scale, multisite demonstration projects demonstrating the cost-effectiveness of the family-centered medical home model.

The Family-Centered Medical Home has been most effective in improving health-care quality for children with special health care needs (CSHCN). Children with special health care needs (CSHCN) are defined as children with "a chronic physical, developmental, behavioral, or emotional condition and who also require health and related services of a type or amount beyond that required by children generally." CSHCN represent less than 15% of all U.S. children, and at least 20% of the children of parents in low-income, low-literacy communities. However, CSCHN are responsible for more than 70% of child health care expenditures.[27,74] Compared with other children, CSHCN have 2.5 times the number of missed school days; experience twice as many unmet health needs; and account for 5 times as many hospital days.[63] Common child chronic conditions include asthma, oral health problems, and behavioral health conditions (including attention deficit hyperactivity disorder), but many CSHCN have rare congenital disorders and multiple comorbid conditions. Among the adults who care for CSHCN, more than 30% have low health literacy.

The children of low-literacy adults are at greatest risk for low health care quality, as measured by health care utilization, health behaviors, and other health outcomes. In studies among children with asthma and type-1 diabetes, those who have caregivers with low health literacy are at increased risk for unmet health care needs, worse control of illness, and more preventable use of the emergency room.[92-95] Adjusted for socioeconomic status and ethnicity, mothers with low health literacy skills are more likely to smoke[96] and to have depressive symptoms.[45-48] Several studies have demonstrated that mothers with low literacy were significantly less likely to understand information regarding home safety for young children.[15,29] Low maternal health literacy is associated with increased risk for child obesity—including a decreased likelihood of exclusive breastfeeding at two months postpartum,[40] decreased ability to understand and use and WIC information,[51] nonuse of nutrition-fact labels when choosing food for their children,[42] and inaccurate perception of child weight.[43]

Parent health literacy may be a critical family-centered characteristic that moderates the effectiveness of the Family-Centered Medical Home—for children with chronic health conditions, for children at risk for chronic-health conditions, and for all children. At the level of state programs, health systems, and individual practices—a Family-Centered Medical Home reform offers ready opportunities to implement both "universal health literacy precautions" and targeted approaches that provide families with limited health literacy a more culturally effective and intensive care coordination to meet their children's health needs.

ACA-Related Recommendations. ACA provides significant opportunities to implement literacy-sensitive approaches to the Family-Centered Medical Home:

1. *Tailor Quality Improvement Efforts for Low-Literacy Families in the Family-Centered Medical Home.* By mandating attention to "consumer health literacy" in the actions of AHRQ's newly established Center for Quality Improvement and Patient Safety, Section 3501 of ACA encourages all federally funded QI efforts to accommodate adults with limited literacy skills, including adults who care for young children. Accountable care organizations (ACOs) should provide child health care coordination that targets low-literacy communities. Public health and health care agencies may be able to use parent literacy skills, alongside other risk adjustment measures, to target enhanced care coordination services. With diminished resources and increased incentives to reduce costs—Medicaid managed care organizations and the new Accountable Care Organizations established by ACA may be able to improve the quality of care for children with complex conditions by tailoring their care-coordination services to match the health literacy skills of their parents. The result may be significant reductions in disparities for children with special health care needs.
2. *Develop Low-Literacy Decision Aids for the Family-Centered Medical Home.* By funding the CDC and the NIH to develop low-literacy decision aids to enhance shared decision making, Section 3506 provides a platform for developing systems that increase parent and child involvement in the care of a child chronic illness. To be effective for child health, these decision aids must be family-centered, with an attention not only to the literacy-needs of parents, but also to the developmentally-appropriate literacy skills of children. One pressing need is to develop, test, and disseminate electronic child health records that are understandable and useful to all stakeholders: children, their parents, their care providers, and their care coordinators.
3. *Test the Cost-Effectiveness of Health Literacy Interventions, through Demonstration Projects for the Family-Centered Medical Home.* In addition to $225 million in CHIPRA demonstration-project funding, ACA funds a new Center for Medicare and Medicaid Innovation (CMI) that will fund quality-improvement demonstration programs in care coordination, as well as additional funds for maternal-infant home visiting programs (Sec. 2951) and childhood obesity demonstration projects (Sec. 4306). Each of these demonstration projects provides an opportunity to integrate and assess the cost-

effectiveness of literacy-sensitive approaches. In addition to the targeted approaches and tools described above, these may include literacy-sensitive tools (and accompanying training for health care and paraprofessional staff) that target high-impact child health outcomes: healthy nutritional and physical activity behaviors, child-safety behaviors, oral health practices, childhood immunizations, interpretation of common child health screening tests, parent mental health, and parent smoking cessation.

3. TO IMPROVE CHILD MEDICATION SAFETY

Medication errors may be more likely in families with limited literacy skills. Interpretation of dosing charts for OTC medicines is significantly more difficult for caregivers with limited literacy or numeracy skills.[30-32, 69] A recent study by Lokker et al demonstrated that at least two in three caregivers considered over-the-counter (OTC) cough and cold medications appropriate for infants, despite viewing package labeling that suggested otherwise; misinterpretation of OTC product age indication was highest among those with the lowest numeracy skills.[33] Other work has demonstrated that multiple reasons for confusion and misdosing of common liquid pediatric medications. Using commonly distributed dosing cups, parents are prone to significant errors in dosing liquid prescription medication. In one study of a common pediatric prescription medication, Yin et al.[30] documented a mean error rate of 48% from the recommended dose. Several investigators have demonstrated the effectiveness of more clearly labeled dosing devices, the use of pictograms, and other low-literacy tools in reducing parent dosing errors.

ACA-Related Recommendations. Section 3507 of the ACA provides specific mandate for the HHS to improve the safe use of medications by adopting and implementing new evidence-based standards for prescription medication labeling. With particular attention to the care of children who rely on liquid medication, the health literacy opportunities include the following:

1. Adopt and enforce standards for dosing instructions for nonprescription pediatric liquid medication.
2. Adopt and enforce standards for dosing instructions for prescription liquid medication.
3. Adopt and enforce standards for the use of safe, easy-to-use dosing devices for liquid medication.

4. TO IMPROVE SKILLS OF THE PEDIATRIC WORKFORCE

Background. Medical providers' ability to address health literacy related communication barriers undergird all of the 6 competencies developed by the American College of Graduate Medical Education (ACGME). These competencies include interpersonal communication, professionalism, practice-based learning, systems-based practice, patient care, and medical knowledge. Nonetheless, the ACGME and the professional bodies that regulate post-graduate training for physicians, physician assistants, and nurse practitioners have no specific requirement to train these providers in evidence-based communication skills.

Among pediatric providers who have completed their post-graduate training, there is a widely recognized sense of incompetency and need for greater training to meet the literacy and language demands of their patients and families. In a recent survey of a nationally representative sample of pediatric providers, more than 75% reported no regular use of evidence-based communication skills—such as employing teach-back conversations, reducing medical jargon, and using drawings or low-literacy texts to enhance verbal communication. Happily, nearly 2 in 3 providers suggested they would be interested in training to help address these deficiencies.

In 2009, the American Academy of Pediatrics launched an interactive, online training module in Health Literacy as part of its PediaLink™ training center. Its brief, actionable pages comply with educational and behavioral theory, and it has been effectively pretested among pediatric trainees. Use of the module nationwide, however, remains minimal. Other similar, evidence-based training modules for internal-medicine physicians and for more general populations of medical providers are also available.

ACA-Related Recommendations. By Amending Title VII of the Public Health Service Act, Section 5301 of the ACA provides HHS the opportunity, mandate, and funding to equip the future physician workforce to address modifiable causes of disparities (especially language and literacy). To realize this goal, the IOM Roundtable on Health Literacy should join HHS, HRSA, and other federal agencies to partner with professional organizations responsible for medical-provider training. Specifically for pediatrics, these include the ACGME, the AAP, the Association of Pediatric Program Directors (APPD), and the National Association of Pediatric Nurse Practitioners (NAPNAP). These agencies and societies should agree to the following:

1. Make health literacy training a required component of post-graduate training in child health (e.g., Pediatrics, Family Medicine, Pediatric Nurse Practitioners)

2. Improve and disseminate evidence-based Health Literacy Training Modules for pediatric providers, trainees, and community providers alike.

Acknowledgment: Thanks to Kartik Telekuntla for his assistance with background research and checking references.

INFORMATION SOURCES

1. U.S. Preventive Services Taskforce, www.thecommunityguide.gov, accessed October 20, 2008.
2. AAP National Center of Medical Home Initiatives for Children with Special Needs, www.medicalhomeinfo.org, accessed March 8, 2009.
3. Hagan JF, Shaw JS, Duncan P. *Bright Futures: Guidelines for Health Supervision of Infants, Children, and Adolescents.* Third Edition. Elk Grove Village, IL: American Academy of Pediatrics; 2008.
4. Scott TL, Gazmararian JA, Williams MV, Baker DW. Health literacy and preventive health care use among Medicare enrollees in a managed care organization. *Med Care.* 2002;40:395-404.
5. Bennett CL, Ferreira MR, Davis TC, et al. Relation between literacy, race, and stage of presentation among low-income patients with prostate cancer. *J Clin Oncol.* 1998;16: 3101-4.
6. Schillinger D, Grumbach K, Piette J, et al. Association of health literacy with diabetes outcomes. *JAMA.* 2002;288:475-82.
7. Rothman RL, Housam R, Weiss H, et al. Patient understanding of food labels: the role of literacy and numeracy. *Am J Prev Med.* 2006;31(5):391-8.
8. Williams MV, Baker DW, Parker RM, Nurss JR. Relationship of functional health literacy to patients' knowledge of their chronic disease. A study of patients with hypertension and diabetes. *Arch Intern Med.* 1998;158:166-72.
9. Battersby C, Hartley K, Fletcher AE, et al. Cognitive function in hypertension: a community based study. *J Hum Hypertens.* 1993;7:117-23.
10. Arnold CL, Davis TC, Berkel HJ, et al. Smoking status, reading level, and knowledge of tobacco effects among low-income pregnant women. *Prev Med.* 2001;32:313-20.
11. Ratzan SC, Parker RM. Introduction. In National Library of Medicine Current Bibliographies in Medicine: Health Literacy. Selden CR, Zorn M, et al., Ed. NLM Pub. No. CBM 2000-1. Bethesda, MD: National Institutes of Health, U.S. Department of Health and Human Services.
12. Nielsen-Bohlman L, Panzer A, Kindig DA. **Health Literacy: A Prescription to End Confusion.** Washington, DC: The National Academies Press; 2004.
13. National Center for Education Statistics, U.S. Department of Education. A First Look at the Literacy of America's Adults in the 21st Century. NCES Publication No. 2006-470.
14. Kutner, M, Greenberg, E, Jin,Y, et al. *The Health Literacy of America's Adults: Results From the 2003 National Assessment of Adult Literacy* (NCES 2006–483). U.S. Department of Education. Washington, DC: National Center for Education Statistics; 2006.
15. Yin HS, Johnson M, Mendelsohn AL, et al. The Health Literacy of Parents in the U.S.: A Nationally Representative Study. *Submitted to Pediatrics (contained in this supplement).*
16. Davis TC, Humiston SG, Arnold CL, et al. Recommendations for effective newborn screening communication: results of focus groups with parents, providers, and experts. *Pediatrics.* 2006;117:S326-40.

17. Arnold CL, Davis TC, Frempong JO, et al. Assessment of newborn screening parent education materials. *Pediatrics* 2006;117(5 Pt 2):S320-5.

18. Farrell M, Deuster L, Donovan J, Christopher S. Jargon during counseling about newborn screening. *Pediatrics* 2008;122:243-50.

19. Sanders L, Federico S, Abrams MA, et al. Readability of enrollment forms for the State Children's Health Insurance Program (SCHIP). Pediatric Academic Societies Annual Meeting, Toronto, Canada, Platform Presentation, 5-8 May 2007.

20. Davis TC, Mayeaux EJ, Fredrickson D, et al. Reading ability of parents compared with reading level of pediatric patient education materials. *Pediatrics.* 1994;93:460-68.

21. Davis TC, Crouch MA, Wills G, et al. The gap between patient reading comprehension and the readability of patient education materials. *J Fam Pract.* 1990;31:533-38.

22. CDS VIS for Polio, accessed May 26, 2007, at http://www.cdc.gov/nip/publications/vis/vis-IPV.txt.

23. Forbes SG, Align A. Poor readability of written asthma management plans found in national guidelines. *Pediatrics.* 2002;109(4):e52.

24. Abrams MA, Dreyer BP, Eds. Plain Language Pediatrics: Health Literacy Strategies and Communication Resources for Common Pediatric Topics. American Academy of Pediatrics: Elk Grove Village, IL; 2009.

25. D'Allesandro DM, Kingsley P, Johnson-West K. The readability of pediatric patient education materials on the world wide web. *Archives of Pediatrics and Adolescent Medicine* 2001;155:807-12.

26. Sanders LM, Lewis J, Brosco JP. Low caregiver health literacy: risk factor for child access to a medical home. Presented at the Pediatric Academic Societies Annual Meeting; May 15, 2005; Washington, DC.

27. Sanders LM, Thompson VT, Wilkinson JD. Caregiver health literacy and the use of child health services. *Pediatrics.* 2007;119(1):86-92.

28. Fredrickson DD, Washington RL, Pham N, et al. Reading grade levels and health behaviors of parents at child clinics. *Kans Med.* 1995;96:127-9.

29. Llewellyn G, McConnell D, Honey A, et al. Promoting health and home safety for children of parents with intellectual disability: a randomized controlled trial. *Res Dev Disabil.* 2003;24:405-31.

30. Yin HS, Dreyer BP, Foltin G, et al. Association of low caregiver health literacy with reported use of nonstandardized dosing instruments and lack of knowledge of weight-based dosing. *Ambul Pediatr.* 2007;7(4):292-8.

31. Wolf MS, Davis TC, Shrank W, et al. To err is human: patient misinterpretations of prescription drug label instructions. *Patient Educ Couns.* 2007;67(3):293-300.

32. Davis TC, Wolf MS, Bass PF, et al. Literacy and misunderstanding prescription drug labels. *Ann Intern Med.* 2006;145(12)887-94.

33. Lokker N, Sanders LM, et al. Misinterpretation of over-the-counter cough and cold medications. Pediatrics. In press 2008.

34. Davis TC, Byrd RS, Arnold CL, et al. Low literacy and violence among adolescents in a summer sports program. *J Adolesc Health.* 1999;24:403-11.

35. Stanton WR, Feehan M, McGee R, Silva PA. The relative value of reading ability and IQ as predictors of teacher-reported behavior problems. *J Learn Disabil.* 1990;23:514-7.

36. McGee R, Prior M, William S, et al. The long-term significance of teacher-rated hyperactivity and reading ability in childhood: findings from two longitudinal studies. *J Child Psychol Psychiatry.* 2002;43(8):1004-17.

37. Miles SB, Stipek D. Contemporaneous and longitudinal associations between social behavior and literacy achievement in a sample of low-income elementary school children. *Child Development.* 2006;77(1);103-17.

38. Hawthorne G. Pre-teenage drug use in Australia: the key predictors and school-based drug education. *J Adolesc Health.* 1997;20:384-95.

39. Fortenberry JD, McFarlane MM, Hennessy M, et al. Relation of health literacy to gonor-rhea related care. *Sex Transm Infect.* 2001;77:206-11.
40. Kaufman H, Skipper B, Small L, et al. Effect of literacy on breast-feeding outcomes. *South Med J.* 2001;94:293-6.
41. Rothman RL, Housam R, Weiss H, et al. Patient understanding of food labels: the role of literacy and numeracy. *Am J Prev Med.* 2006;31:391-8.
42. Kyvelos E, Mendelsohn AL, Tomopoulos S, et al. Use of Food Labels by Low Socioeco-nomic Status (SES) Parents: Associations with Material Hardship and Health Literacy. *Pediatric Academic Societies' Meeting.* May 2008, Honolulu, HI E-PAS2008:635811.10.
43. Yin HS, Dreyer BP, van Schaick L, et al. Factors associated with overweight status in low SES children: role of parent health literacy. *Pediatric Academic Societies' Meeting.* May 2008, Honolulu, HI. E-PAS2008:634474.49.
44. Arnold CL, Davis TC, Berkel HJ, Jet al. Smoking status, reading level, and knowledge of tobacco effects among low-income pregnant women. *Prev Med.* 2001;32:313-20.
45. Weiss BD, Francis L, Senf JH, et al. Literacy education as treatment for depression in patients with limited literacy and depression: a randomized controlled trial. *J Gen Intern Med.* 2006;21(8):823-8.
46. Bennett I, Switzer J, Aguirre A, et al. "Breaking it down": patient-clinician communica-tion and prenatal care among African American women of low and higher literacy. *Ann Fam Med.* 2006;4(4):334-40.
47. Sanders LM, Shone LP, Conn KM, et al. Parent depression and low health literacy: risk factors for child health disparities? *Pediatric Academic Societies Annual Meeting,* Toronto, Canada, 5-8 May 2007.
48. Poresky RH, Daniels AM. Two-year comparison of income, education, and depression among parents participating in regular Head Start or supplementary Family Service Center Services. *Psychol Rep.* 2001;88:787-96.
49. Bandura, A. Social Learning Theory. New York: General Learning Press; 1977.
50. Berwick D. Eleven worthy aims for clinical leadership of health system reform. *JAMA.* 1994;272(10):797-805.
51. Newes-Adeyi G, Helitzer DL, Roter D, Caulfield LE. Improving client-provider com-munication: evaluation of a training program for women, infants and children (WIC) professionals in New York state. *Patient Educ Couns.* 2004;55(2):210-7.
52. Williams MV, Davis TC, Parker RM, Weiss BD. The role of health literacy in patient-physician communication. *Fam Med.* 2002;34:383-89.
53. Whitlock ER, Qrleans CT, Pender N, Allan J. Evaluating primary care behavioral coun-seling interventions: an evidence-based approach. *Am J Prev Med.* 2002;22:267-84.
54. Towle A, Godolphin W. Framework for teaching and learning informed shared decision making. *BMJ* 1999; 319(7212):766-71.
55. Flowers L. Teach-back improves informed consent. *OR Manager.* 2006;22(3):25-6.
56. Mayeaux EJ Jr, Murphy PW, Arnold C, et al. Improving patient education for patients with low literacy skills. *Am Fam Physician.* 1996;53(1):205-11.
57. Mellins RB, Evans D, Clark N, et al. Developing and communicating a long-term treat-ment plan for asthma. *Am Fam Physician.* 2000;61(8):2419-28, 2433-4.
58. Rider EA, Keefer CH. Communication skills competencies: definitions and a teaching toolbox. *Med Educ.* 2006;40(7):624-9.
59. Kripalani S, Robertson R, Love-Ghaffari MH, et al. Development of an illustrated medication schedule as a low-literacy patient education tool. *Patient Educ Couns.* 2007;66(3):368-77.
60. Wolff K, Cavanaugh K, Malone R, et al. The diabetes literacy and numeracy education toolkit (DLNET): materials to facilitate diabetes education and management in patients with low literacy and numeracy skills. *Diabetes Education.* 2009;35(2):233-45.

61. Dunn RA, Shenouda PE, Martin DR, Schultz AJ. Videotape increases parent knowledge about poliovirus vaccines and choices of polio vaccination schedules. *Pediatrics*. 1998;102,e26.

62. Masley S, Sokoloff J, Hawes C. Planning group visits for high-risk patients. *Fam Pract Manag*. 2000;7(6):33-7.

63. Houck S, Kilo C, Scott JC. Improving patient care. Group visits 101. *Fam Pract Manag*. 2003;10(5):66-8.

64. Bunik M, Glazner JE, Chandramouli V, et al. Pediatric telephone call centers: how do they affect health care use and costs? *Pediatrics*. 2007;119(2):e305-13.

65. Gielen AC, McKenzie LB, McDonald EM, et al. Using a computer kiosk to promote child safety: results of a randomized, controlled trial in an urban pediatric emergency department. *Pediatrics* 2007;120(2):330-9.

66. Davis TC, Fredrickson DD, Bocchini C, et al. Improving vaccine risk/benefit communication with an immunization education package: a pilot study. *Ambul Pediatr*. 2000;2(3):193-200.

67. Edwards A, Elwyn G, Mulley A. Explaining risks: turning numerical data into meaningful pictures. *BMJ*. 2002;324(7341):827-30.

68. Rand CM, Conn KM, Crittenden CN, Halterman JS. Does a color-coded method for measuring acetaminophen doses reduce the likelihood of dosing error? *Arch Pediatr Adolesc Med*. 2004;158(7):625-7.

69. Frush KS, Luo X, Hutchinson P, Higgins JN. Evaluation of a method to reduce over-the-counter medication dosing error. *Arch Pediatr Adolesc Med*. 2004;158(7):620-4.

70. Doak CC, Doak LG, Root JH. Teaching Patients with Low Literacy Skills, 2nd ed., Philadelphia: Lippincott; 1996.

71. Davis TC, Gazmararian J, Kennen EM. Approaches to improving health literacy: lessons from the field. *J Health Commun*. 2006;11(6):551-4.

72. Rich M. Health literacy via media literacy: video intervention/prevention assessment. *American Behavioral Scientist*. 2004;48(2):165-88.

73. Cooley WC, McAllister JW, Sherrieb K, Clark RE. The Medical Home Index: development and validation of a new practice-level measure of implementation of the Medical Home model. *Ambul Pediatr*. 2003;3(4):173-80.

74. Shaller D. Implementing and using quality measures for children's health care: perspectives on the state of the practice. *Pediatrics*. 2004;113(1 Pt 2):217-27.

75. National Health Education Standards PreK-12. 2nd ed. American Cancer Society. 2007.

76. Marx E, Hudson N, Deal TB, et al. Promoting health literacy through the health education assessment project. *J Sch Health*. 2007;77:157-63.

77. Golbeck AL, Ahlers-Schmidt CR, Paschal AM. Health Literacy and Adult Basic Education Assessments. *Adult Basic Education: An Interdisciplinary Journal for Adult Literacy Educational Planning*. 2005(15):151-68.

78. Kropsky JA, Keckly PH, Jensen PL. School-based obesity prevention programs: an evidence-based review. *Obesity*. 2008;16(5):1009-18.

79. Flynn BS, Worden JK, Secker-Walker RH, et al. Prevention of cigarette-smoking through mass-media intervention and school programs. *Am J Publ Health*. 1992;82(6):827-34.

80. Kolbe L, Kann L, Patterson B, et al. Enabling the nation's schools to help prevent heart disease, stroke, cancer, COPD, diabetes, and other serious health problems. *Pub Health Rep*. 2004;119(3):286-302.

81. Kann L, Brener N, Wechsler H. Overview and summary: School Health Policies and Programs Study 2006. *J Sch Health*. 2007;77(8):385-97.

82. Wagner EH, Austin BT, Von Korff M. Organizing care for patients with chronic illness. *Milbank Q*. 1996;74(4):511-44.

83. Halfon N, DuPlessis N, Inkelas M. Transforming the U.S. Child Health System. *Health Affairs*. March/April 2007;26(2):315-29.

84. Arah OA, Westert GP, Hurst J, Klazing NS. A conceptual framework for the OECD Health Care Quality Indicators Project. *Int J Qual Health Care.* 2006;18 Suppl 1:5-13.

85. Wagner EH. Chronic disease management: What will it take to improve care for chronic illness? *Effective Clinical Practice.* 1998;1(1):2-4.

86. Chew D, Bradley KA, Boyko EJ. Brief questions to identify patients with inadequate health literacy. *Fam Med.* 2004;36(8):588-94.

87. Parker RM, Baker DW, Williams MV, Nurss JR. The test of functional health literacy in adults: a new instrument for measuring patients' literacy skills. *Journal of General Internal Medicine* 1995; 10(10):537-41.

88. Nurss J. Difficulties in Functional Health Literacy Screening in Spanish-Speaking Adults. *Journal of Reading* 1995;38(8):32-37.

89. Davis TC, Long SW, Jackson RH, et al. Rapid estimate of adult literacy in medicine: a shortened screening instrument. *Fam Med* 1993;25(6):391-5.

90. Lee SY, Bender DE, Ruiz RE, Cho YI. Development of an easy-to-use Spanish health literacy test. *Health Serv Res.* 2006;41(4 Pt 1):1392-412.

91. Institute of Medicine. Unequal Treatment: Confronting Racial and Ethnic Disparities in Health Care. Washington, DC: National Academies Press; 2003.

92. Wittich AR, Mangan J, Grad R, et al. Pediatric Asthma: Caregiver Health Literacy and the Clinician's Perception. Journal of Asthma 2007; 44(1):51-5.

93. Schillinger D, Barton LR, Karter AJ, et al. Does literacy mediate the relationship between education and health outcomes? A study of a low-income population with diabetes. *Public Health Reports.* 2006;121(3):245-54.

94. Sanders LM, Rothman R, Franco V, et al. Low Parent Health Literacy is Associated with Poor Glycemic Control in Children with Type 1 Diabetes Mellitus. Pediatric Academic Societies Meeting, Honolulu, May 2008

95. DeWalt DA, Dilling MH, Rosenthal MS, Pignone MP. Low parental literacy is associated with worse asthma care measures in children. *Ambul Pediatr.* 2007;7:25-31.

96. Arnold CL, Davis TC, Berkel HJ. Smoking status, reading level, and knowledge of tobacco effects among low-income pregnant women. *Prev Med.* 2001;32:313-20.

97. Institute of Medicine. Priority Areas for National Action: Transforming Health Care Quality. K Adams and J.M. Corrigan. Washington, DC: The National Academies Press; 2003.